Miasms as Practical Tools

A Homeopathic Approach to Chronic Disease

John Saxton
BVetMed, VetFFHom, CertIAVH, MRCVS

BEACONSFIELD PUBLISHERS LTD
Beaconsfield, Bucks, UK

First published 2006

email: books@beaconsfield-publishers.co.uk
Website: www.beaconsfield-publishers.co.uk

British Library Cataloguing in Publication Data

Saxton, John
Miasms as practical tools: a homeopathic approach to chronic disease. – (The Beaconsfield homeopathic library; no. 25)
1. Chronic diseases – Homeopathic treatment
2. Homeopathy – Materia medica and therapeutics
I. Title
615.5′32
ISBN–10: 0–906584–58–2

Phototypeset by Gem Graphics, Trenance, Mawgan Porth, Cornwall
in 10 on 12¼ Times.
Printed and bound in Great Britain at The Alden Press, Oxford

Acknowledgements

My sincere thanks to Sue Armstrong, Nick Churchill, Dr David Curtin, Dr Linda Johnston, Dee MacLachlan, Francis Treuherz and Elaine Walker, each of whom at some stage read a draft of the work and made many very helpful comments, all of which I have been glad to be able to take into account when preparing the final version. My thanks also to my many colleagues of all medical disciplines worldwide, whose convivial and unguarded observations have added much to the development of my ideas and who thus have contributed, both knowingly and unknowingly, to this book.

Above all, my deepest thanks go to my wife Pat for her unfailing encouragement, understanding and helpful advice, as well as for introducing me to homeopathy in the first place.

J.S.

Preface

The subject of miasms is a perplexing one, and from the earliest days their place in the homeopathic view of chronic disease has created controversy. There are some homeopaths who have doubts about the relevance of the basic concept, and others who reject the theory entirely. Still others, while accepting the reality of the forces, are doubtful about their role in practical prescribing. Some practitioners are building new philosophical layers onto the original concepts in an attempt to understand better the full extent of their dynamics. For many people starting out on the homeopathic route, all of this can cause confusion.

The purpose of this book is not to rehearse in detail the arguments concerning the very existence of miasms, as the underlying premise of the work is that these influences do exist. The aim is to provide a possible theoretical framework within which the reader can develop their ideas and understanding of what many regard as a central feature of homeopathy. It is hoped too that those with a deeper knowledge of the subject of miasms will also find something of value here, enabling them to acquire a different perspective on the subject.

In modern Western societies chronic disease is now the main enemy, as opposed to the acute epidemics of the past. Hahnemann's view of chronic disease and his concept of miasms provide insights into the understanding and relief of these conditions. Above all, the concept of miasms is a practical therapeutic tool and its use as such will enhance prescribing skills. It is hoped that after reading this book practitioners will be able to apply the concepts more effectively for the benefit of their patients, human or animal. A basic knowledge of homeopathic principles and practice is assumed, and the 6th edition of the *Organon*, edited by Wenda Brewster O'Reilly, has been used as the principal source throughout.

The book presents the author's personal understanding of the concept of miasms as it works for him. The cases quoted are not designed to show that the miasmatic approach is necessarily uppermost in every prescribing situation, but rather that a miasmatic pattern can be seen to run through every case. Inevitably the author's veterinary background and experience have been a major influence in the approach, but the ideas are not confined, or only applicable, to the animal world. The principles are basic to homeopathy and can be applied to the human situation just as much as to the animal. The problems of chronic disease are common to all species. Anything that contributes to the understanding of those problems will be helpful, and it is in that context that this work is offered.

Contents

Chapter 1

The Historical Perspective

The Original Ideas

Homeopathy is portrayed sometimes, even by those who practice it, as simply a different system of treatment, whereas in reality there is much more to it than just using different therapeutic agents. Homeopathy has at its heart a very different approach to health compared to other systems, and in disease this is utilised to work with the body's own healing potential rather than opposing and weakening its inherent vitality. As such it is a radical departure from the current orthodox way of thinking. Conventional treatments of both the allopathic type, where there is no dynamic relationship between the disease and the therapy, and the antipathic form with its direct antagonism to the disease dynamic, can weaken the natural resilience of the patient.

The widening application of homeopathy's basic ideas has resulted in an accentuation of the philosophical differences between the systems. These differences stem from the sharply contrasting views of the true cause of illness and how the mind and body function in both health and disease, and it is in this context that Hahnemann's concept of chronic disease is so important. His complete disillusionment with the conventional medicine of his day arose as a result of his frustration as a clinician with his inability to cure his patients, including members of his own family. More than that, he became convinced that in many cases it was the harmful effects of existing treatments that contributed in large part to the death or continuing poor health of the patient. However, although he ceased to practise as a result of this frustration, his thoughts still remained with the problems of healing and the mode of action of medicines. Even as a translator, to which activity he turned as a means of earning a living, he still retained his links with the medical world and continued to produce original scientific texts, as well as examining and commenting on the work of others.

In 1789 he published a major article on venereal disease, *Instructions for Surgeons Respecting Venereal Disease,* in which he put forward ideas regarding the mode of action of mercury that even then were moving towards the homeopathic concept. Already there were indications in his writing of ideas, particularly concerning the inappropriateness of local treatment, that were later to be incorporated into the miasmatic theory. This was in contradistinction to a body of medical opinion at the time, which held that venereal disease could only be cured by the complete elimination of the local symptoms. Hahnemann's thoughts along this and other lines culminated in his rejection of the explanation of the action of cinchona bark (quinine) in Marsh Fever (malaria), which he came across whilst translating Cullen's *Treatise on Materia Medica* in 1790. His subsequent experiment with cinchona in the same year led to his final understanding of the true mode of action and to his formulation of the basic concept of homeopathy. In 1796 he published his *Essay on a new principle for ascertaining the curative powers of drugs, with a few glances at those hitherto employed*, in which he outlined his first thoughts on this new method of healing and the new way of ascertaining the true therapeutic effects of medicines.

The value of this new method and the soundness of its principles were soon established, and he and his followers subsequently added a steady stream of new remedies to their range of therapeutic agents. Further observation and thought followed, and finally, in 1805, he published *The Medicine of Experience*. This contained the essentials of his thinking, which five years later was expanded into the first edition of the *Organon*, published in 1810.

Concepts of Chronic Disease

Despite the early success of the new method, homeopathy in practice did not always live up to the early and very high expectations that Hahnemann had of it, either from the theoretical point of view or from the response seen in individual cases. It had certainly proved its worth in cases of acute disease, but he and his followers were still encountering many other intractable cases, and in spite of the increasing number of remedies and the developing skills of those doctors who espoused the homeopathic method, these were not being permanently resolved. Complete cures were indeed being obtained by using homeopathy where the other methods of the time were failing, but not in every case, and all concerned felt that in those instances their results could be better. Some of his followers believed that the only difficulty lay in the still small number of remedies at their disposal, and that over time and with more new remedies the problem would in effect solve itself. Hahnemann did not believe this, because in spite of the regular addition of new remedies and the consequent improvements in treatment and case management, the position with regard to these intractable diseases did not change.

He considered that there must be some other explanation. In the first chapter of his great work, *The Chronic Diseases: Their Peculiar Nature and Their Homeopathic Cure,* first published in 1828, he wrote: 'The followers of Homeopathy have hitherto thus consoled themselves; but this excuse or so-called consolation (i.e. not enough remedies), never satisfied the founder of Homeopathy – particularly because even the new additions of proved valuable medicines, increasing from year to year, have not advanced the healing of chronic disease by a single step.'

A very great number of remedies have entered the materia medica since Hahnemann's time, and the total continues to increase. New insights into understanding them, and hence into prescribing approaches, have been developed and further improvements in hygiene and public health have occurred over the same time. In spite of these developments, the problems associated with the cure of chronic disease are today still far from being satisfactorily solved.

Hahnemann's answer to these problems was the theory of miasms. He started from the view that the vital force was essentially the means whereby the body maintained what he described as 'the unimpeded progress of life'. In all but the simplest cases this was unable to overcome challenges and restore normal health without help. Well-selected homeopathic remedies could provide that help. Even in severe acute disease it had been shown that the vital force, with the correct stimulation, was capable of responding to the disease situation and recreating health. Why was the same vital force, with the same correct stimulation, not able to overcome these other diseases in the same way?

Between 1816 and 1817 he had realised that the key to chronic disease was to be found in the solution of that problem. In an article on the treatment of venereal disease, published in 1816 – *On the venereal disease and its ordinary improper treatment* – he makes a clear connection between the improper treatment of skin disease, characterised as the 'itch', and the subsequent development of internal disease. His work over the next twelve years provided him with what he regarded as the complete answer and led to the publication of *The Chronic Diseases.*

The 'failures' in these chronic cases showed themselves in one of two ways. Firstly, the apparent resolution of a seemingly acute condition which would then reappear some time later, possibly in a more virulent form. Secondly, the resolution of a particular presenting problem would restore health for a short time, but the patient would then develop the syndrome of an apparently different disease. Remedies that had proved effective in similar cases, and which were still indicated, failed to produce the desired results. Further homeopathic treatment with other remedies could be met with further apparent success but the pattern of recurring illness would frequently, although not inevitably, repeat itself.

The theory of miasms accounts for these observations by postulating an interference with the normal healing processes of the body, due to influences that block its normal responses to the disease condition. At first sight this appeared to suggest that specific external agents became so integrated into the body's make-up as to permanently affect its function and that these could not then be removed, even by the most intensive and prolonged courses of treatment. First and foremost was the concept of psora, which Hahnemann called 'the mother of all disease', and which he claimed was so diffuse and widespread as to account for seven-eighths of all illness – in fact virtually any condition other than the venereal diseases. He traced its origins from almost prehistoric times, claiming that its manifestations had changed over the years but that they were always linked to the appearance at some stage of an eruption on the skin.

The venereal diseases gonorrhoea and syphilis were included as representing the two other basic causes of chronic disease. Conventional treatment, of course, played its part in weakening the patient and further aggravating the conditions. Apart from the general weakening effect due to the toxic nature of many conventional medicines of the time, the other major effect was due to the concentration by physicians on the removal of the external manifestations of disease, thereby deepening the level at which the disease subsequently appeared. In Paragraph 203 of the *Organon* Hahnemann states: 'Every external treatment for clearing away such local symptoms from the surface of the body, without having cured the internal miasmatic disease … has become the most prevalent source of all the countless named and unnamed chronic sufferings under which humanity so generally sighs.' Similarly in Paragraph 204, which marks the start of his detailed discussion of chronic disease and the miasms, he says: 'If, by external means, these miasms are robbed of their representative local symptoms (which allay the general suffering), sooner or later the characteristic diseases that the Originator of Nature has appointed for each of the miasms must inevitably unfold and erupt.'

Reactions to the Theory

The new theory split the developing homeopathic world, and in some ways the arguments continue to the present day. Hahnemann realised the controversy that his ideas would generate, writing to Drs Stapf and Gross in 1827 that 'it will take them (his followers) six months to recover from the shock, and another six months to begin to understand.' Eight hundred unsold copies of the first edition had to be scrapped as 'worthless paper', leading to a claim from his publisher for recompense. In spite of this, a second edition was published in 1835.

There were those who believed that, although they could not grasp the full implications of Hahnemann's ideas, if the master had said it was so, then so it must be. However imperfectly, they attempted to put the new ideas into practice and wrote with enthusiasm about the theory and their results. Others were more cautious, taking the stance that while the basic homeopathic philosophy was correct and had been proved in practice, this concept was a step too far. They accordingly continued to practise as they had always been doing, taking no account of the new concepts. Even Hering (1800–1880), certainly one of the most enthusiastic of Hahnemann's disciples, at one time questioned the relevance of the theory, maintaining that the Law of Similars was all that was required for successful prescribing. His initial view, as stated in his introduction to the American edition of the *Organon* in 1836, was: 'What important influence can it exert whether a homeopath adopt the theoretical opinions of Hahnemann [on chronic disease] or not, so long as he holds the principal tools of the master and the materia medica of our schools. What influence can it have, whether a physician adopt or reject the psoric theory, so long as he always selects the most similar medicine possible?'

He later came to realise the importance of the miasmatic approach, writing in support of antipsoric remedies in an introduction to the 1845 printing of *The Chronic Diseases*, and also writing of the importance of antipsoric remedies in the treatment of leprosy. J.H. Allen (1854–1925) spelled out the case for the theory in his book *The Chronic Miasms,* published in 1908: 'that such knowledge [of miasms] is the difference between intelligent warfare and fighting in the dark, as what we can see and hear from our patients is only some small fragment of a deep-seated disease.' He also highlighted Hering's insistence on 'the most similar medicine possible' by stating: 'The fact is, we cannot select the most similar remedy possible unless we understand the phenomena of the active and basic miasms; for the true simillimum is always based upon the existing basic miasms, whether we be conscious or unconscious of the fact.' Also in *The Chronic Miasms* he stated that 'the character of the miasm gives us the character of the affectation or the disease formula.'

A third group considered that if this was where homeopathy was leading then it must all be false, and returned to their old ways.

Hahnemann, however, continued to incorporate and expand his ideas and methods. By the time he was practising in Paris at the end of his life (1835–1843), miasmatic considerations formed a large, if not the major, part of his approach, and his writings, particularly the later editions of the *Organon*, reflected this. However, there was a considerable delay in the publication of the Sixth edition, together with his later case notes, partly due to copyright considerations, and partly due to the concerns of his second wife, Mélanie, over the reception of his later ideas. The case notes show a general tendency to start every case with a major miasmatic remedy (usually Sulphur), and then to prescribe again based on the picture that emerged. There was also an increasing use of the new potency scale based on a dilution of one in fifty thousand, which Hahnemann had developed and which he subsequently introduced in the Sixth edition – the so-called LM, or more accurately, Q potencies.

The Sixth edition of the *Organon* was not published in its final form until 1921, which meant that the ideas regarding homeopathic philosophy that were being developed by others throughout the nineteenth and early twentieth centuries, particularly in America, were produced without the influence of Hahnemann's final thoughts. This was unfortunate, as the leap made between the Fifth and Sixth editions was greater than the changes and progressions which had occurred from the First to the Fifth, and represented an important development in the theory and practice of homeopathy. Hahnemann himself described the theory of miasms as a 'keystone' of homeopathy, and the Sixth edition represents his final thoughts on it.

The Clinical Context

It is important to remember the context in which Hahnemann produced his ideas. In spite of his revolutionary approach he was still a product of his time, and his initial training and early experiences greatly influenced his thoughts. From the times of the ancient Egyptians and Greeks, early ideas and observations moving towards concepts broadly similar to those on which he based his theory were known. Further questioning and conclusions can be found in the writings originating from the conventional medical world, both during and prior to his lifetime, some of which he acknowledged. During his lifetime doctors such as Alexander, Leith and Munro in Scotland, and Haller and Crumpe in Germany, were voicing ideas about the size of the necessary dose and the need to know the full effects of the medicines being employed. Even Cullen, although Hahnemann disagreed with him over cinchona and Marsh Fever, had a positive influence in shaping his overall views.

Above all, Hahnemann thought and spoke within the context of the medical language and clinical experience of his time, not only as a means of rationalising and progressing his ideas, but also as a means of communicating with his professional colleagues. It is true that many of those conventional colleagues did not wish to hear what he had to say and rejected his ideas. But for those who did listen it was essential to remain within bounds that they could mutually understand, while at the same time pushing those bounds ever wider.

It is perhaps unfortunate for the understanding of homeopathy generally that much of the original terminology, which was common to all medicine at that time, has been retained. The gigantic strides that have been made in medicine over the past hundred years have altered the conventional language almost beyond recognition. New terms have evolved to describe new concepts, and the relationship of homeopathy to the mainstream of conventional thought has meant that in many ways the gulf has widened. It is possible that the great homeopaths of the nineteenth and twentieth centuries maintained the old terminology partly as a means of emphasising the differences between the systems. In addition, as the conventional approach has become more materialistic there are often no common terms to describe the more spiritual aspects of homeopathic philosophy, or indeed many modern homeopathic concepts generally.

However that may be, behind the language are some profound and significant perceptions. It is interesting to note that some of the ideas now emerging in conventional medicine appear to be moving back towards the concepts that Hahnemann was trying to express in the clinical language of his era. The question is sometimes asked, 'Can a nearly two-hundred-year-old concept be a practical working tool nowadays?' But that concept is as valid today as it was when it was first introduced, because it is based on a thorough understanding of the way that the mind and body function in both health and disease. That understanding was reached as a result of much study and the bringing together of ideas on health and disease from many sources and societies, confirmed by painstaking observation and experimentation over many years. Increasingly, Hahnemann's basic ideas are being shown to be sound, not only in the fields of physiological and basic research (Bellavite and Signorini, 2002) but also in the clinical setting. Modern developments in the field of genetics are equating with the failures of development and function that are the essence of psora, and research and experience with the treatment of conditions such as asthma are confirming what homeopathy understands as the miasmatic nature of the condition. It is reasonable to suggest that it is the conventional world, approaching the subject from an entirely different perspective, which is now adapting its views and coming more into line with Hahnemann's concepts.

Terminology and Development

The first obstacle to be overcome is the term 'miasm' itself. In Hahnemann's day it generally meant some form of noxious substance or influence, the exact nature of which was unknown, but which was recognised to be capable of causing disease. In modern general dictionaries this is still the basis of the definition. It comes from the Greek word *miasma*, meaning pollution, and also from the verb *miainein*, meaning to stain or pollute.

About eighty years before the work of Koch (1843–1910) and Pasteur (1822–1895), towards the end of the nineteenth century and the appearance of germ theory, Hahnemann was using the term in the sense of what would now be recognised as an infectious agent. His writings in relation to cholera and what was then known as Ship Fever reflect this. In modern terminology this was probably a multifactorial acute infection. Even today there is an echo of this use of the term in the concept of an 'acute' miasm, which is in fact not a true chronic miasm at all but rather represents the body's normal reaction to an acute challenge. It is ironic that while Hahnemann was breaking new ground and challenging the whole basis of medical thought, this very inspired leap in one direction was expressed in the accepted terminology of his time, and the continued use of that terminology has hindered the understanding of the theory of miasms ever since.

But without the diagnostic niceties available today, and with the prominent place that scabies, gonorrhoea and syphilis had in the clinical experience of all doctors of that time, it is perhaps not surprising that this became the framework for his new ideas. It was on the effects of what he saw as the inappropriate treatment of these diseases that Hahnemann built his ideas. He realised that the long-term consequences of these treatments varied depending on the disease that had been suffered rather than on the treatment that had been given. Hence the apparent connection was established between the disease and the consequence, although in truth the treatment was the real culprit. As mentioned above, one of his major works prior to homeopathy had been a treatise on venereal disease, and even then he was aware of, and discussed, the harmful effects resulting from suppression of the chancre.

His early thoughts on the development of chronic disease appear at first glance to link the process to what would now be called an infection. The close identification of the sycotic and syphilitic miasms with the venereal diseases, and his historical description of the progress of psora through the ages, initially reinforced that impression. But a closer look at his writings will show that while beginning to recognise the existence of what is now described as infection, he envisaged something more than that right from the outset. In *The Chronic Diseases*, when discussing their true nature, he stresses that what has appeared as psora is the result of conditions being 'medically treated in the worst and most injurious manner'. However, the impression of the contagious nature of the miasmatic forces was nevertheless given, and this has influenced the discussion of the subject of miasms ever since. Based on that impression, many objections have been raised concerning the apparently changing pattern of psora over time and the resulting claim of its almost universal implication in every disease entity. Unfortunately, these objections have been used to question the whole theory of miasms in relation to chronic disease.

But this is to minimise and misunderstand Hahnemann's original concepts. It is clear from his works that from the very start he had a broader vision of the 'pollutant' being more than just an infectious agent, and was concerned rather with the functional reactions of the mind and body than just with the challenging entity. He also considered the attempts of the conventional world to deal with infections in relation to that function, and found them wanting. Long before Pasteur and his final acknowledgement that 'the soil is everything', Hahnemann had reached that same conclusion. Pasteur came to consider that disease could not be fully understood without understanding the individual. He believed that the body's biochemical and physiological state, as well as the person's emotional and mental state, profoundly influenced the course and outcome of disease. It is unfortunate that this part of Pasteur's work has been played down and that a narrower concept of it has been applied in the interpretation of germ theory. It is with the quality of the 'soil' that the theory of miasms is concerned, and indeed Paragraph 2 of the *Organon* emphasises the importance of 'the lifting and annihilation of the disease in its entire extent'. This, of course, implies more than just dealing with the presenting picture of disease.

In addition to these confusions, miasmatic theory is often invoked as a means of explaining the failure of indicated remedies to act, and a miasm is therefore regarded as a block to obtaining a cure. In reality, the theory's purpose is actually one of securing a permanent improvement in the patient's condition. At times Hahnemann does indeed portray the miasms as negative forces capable of both producing and maintaining disease (*Organon*, Paragraphs 79 and 80). But it is vital to realise that the true clinical value of the theory is to provide a way round the obstacles encountered in chronic disease. Once this is appreciated, it is then possible to utilise the theory as a valuable therapeutic tool.

The development of homeopathy in America by Kent (1849–1916) and his colleagues, and the prominence that their ideas attained, has also affected attitudes to the miasmatic theory. Some of them were greatly influenced by the teachings of Swedenborg (1688–1772), the Swedish scientist turned theologian, and his individualistic interpretation of Christian teaching, especially his concept that every physical manifestation has a spiritual equivalent. Kent and William Boericke were both followers of his teachings and this resulted in the introduction of more mystical, esoteric and religious elements into homeopathic thought. Linked to the existing connection with the venereal diseases, which Kent reinforced, this led them to a 'wages of sin' approach, and psora was in some quarters equated with the concept of Original Sin as found in the Judaeo-Christian tradition. Kent, in his *Lectures on Homoeopathic Philosophy*, described psora as 'the very primitive wrong of the human race' and a 'spiritual sickness', and also talked of patients being 'black with syphilis', with the moral implications and condemnation that such statements implied.

Overall, the introduction of a more spiritual dimension, arising in large part from the Swedenborg influence, benefited homeopathy. The dominance of the American ideas over the more pathological approach of Hughes and his English colleagues resulted in a broader-based materia medica and reinforced Hahnemann's ideas on the importance of mental symptoms. Unfortunately, the moral overtones of the American ideas were less helpful to the concept of the miasms. P.N. Banerjee, writing in 1931 (*Chronic Disease – its Cause and Cure*) describes psora as 'a condition of the physical body brought on by evil thinking', and then contrasts sycosis and syphilis with this, these latter two originating from bad and evil action.

Modern Interpretations

Although scabies is potentially found in all species, it is only in humans that gonorrhoea and syphilis are seen as clinical entities. Yet miasmatic influences are as important a consideration in animals as they are in humans.

Modern ideas on the miasms are moving to different understandings and interpretations from those of the nineteenth and early twentieth century. Although initially some of these may seem to contradict Hahnemann's ideas, his original approach of viewing the situations from the functional and dynamic aspect is once more coming to the fore. A strong tradition of miasms in South America (notably Ortega, Toledo, Proceso and Paschero) recognises that the close connection with the venereal infections is misleading, and regards the miasms as being the ultimate cause of disease – the so-called *causa causarum*. They are what make up the 'terrain' on which all challenges impinge. The miasmatic make-up of an individual is considered to be an integral part of the constitutional picture, and may be a block to the true nature and function of that individual. It is the struggle against this miasmatic block which results in the appearance of the particular symptoms seen in an individual case.

Miasms are often regarded as deep-seated predispositions to certain specific diseases. Although this is true it is not the whole story. They are also predispositions to particular ways in which individuals express all disease, no matter what its origin. These expressions will be on all levels of function, from the physical to the higher mental planes. Different species may predominantly exhibit different aspects of the miasmatic picture, although this may in part be a reflection of the prescriber's ability to identify the symptoms presented, particularly in the non-verbal patient. However, each individual miasm appears to influence every species in essentially the same way, depending on the intrinsic nature of the miasm involved.

Over the years the concept of newer miasms in addition to the original three has been developed, and new philosophical interpretations are appearing. In the early part of the twentieth century a clinical pattern was recognised which was classed as the tubercular miasm. Although cancer as a disease has been known for thousands of years, it was not until the second half of the nineteenth century that homeopaths began to recognise a clinical pattern linked to it, which has been called the cancer miasm. There is now talk of an Aids miasm. In recent times Sankaran, the renowned Indian homeopath, has used the theory to interpret and classify the stages of the disease process. New protocols for treatment that use the ideas behind the miasms are being developed.

Although the theory may be regarded primarily as a model to explain certain observed clinical patterns, it is not merely an academic nicety but a practical philosophy that is of daily use in the consulting room. The miasmatic approach to case management offers new perspectives, often revealing the underlying traits and patterns that have produced a particular clinical situation. It is an aid to remedy selection and adds useful information in the search for the simillimum. The interpretation of a case as it develops is made clearer by considering the miasmatic influences, not only by explaining what has happened, but also by indicating the way forward towards cure. The theory of miasms is, above all, a practical doctrine that was developed as a working tool to explain and overcome clinical obstacles.

Chapter 2

The Body in Health and Disease

Normal Physiological Function

The concept that miasms are deep-seated predispositions to disease and disease patterns implies that they have an intimate involvement with the regular functioning of the body. Hence, before looking at miasms in detail it is necessary to consider the normal physiological processes that occur in the everyday process of maintaining and furthering life. These may be divided broadly into three types of function. Conventionally, many different physiological processes are described, but all can be classified generally into one of these three fundamental types, and in the consideration of miasms it must be remembered that the emphasis is on dynamic forces and functions and not on physiological detail.

Firstly, there is the creation of new cells and tissues to replace worn-out or damaged components. There is also the increase in the production of various specialist cells, plus chemical compounds such as hormones, to meet specific requirements. This is seen, for example, in the temporary rise in white blood cells that is generated to deal with an acute infection. The reproductive function is another situation, in some ways the most extreme, where there is the need to increase cell production in face of a particular medium-term physiological need, namely the development of the foetus.

Secondly, there is a functional need to eliminate damaged or obsolete cells and cell products, and to destroy and remove foreign biological invaders and other challenges to the integrity of the body.

Finally, there is the need to ensure the proper internal environment in which the beneficial effects of all the activities can be utilised. This brings into play all the biofeedback and other self-regulatory mechanisms involved in the day-to-day maintenance of health. This implies the monitoring and appropriate adjustment of the rate of production of cells and cell products, which can be considered as a form of control. It is not, of course, control in the sense of 'Do what I tell you when I tell you', but rather much more subtle autogenous regulation. It may be considered, in the modern parlance, as being the role of a group facilitator as opposed to that of the chairman of a meeting.

All these activities and processes go on continuously at both a cellular and biochemical level to create and preserve the harmonious yet dynamic state that is recognised as homeostasis. Renato Azambuja (2004), in a commentary on Maturana's theory of autopoiese [homeostasis], describes this as: 'Living beings are systems that operate in a closed but dynamic relationship of internal states, each with its own sphere of action. For a living being to stay alive the only necessary condition is that its systems continually adjust to the outside environment.' [Author's translation]

Balance as a Prerequisite

In any situation, whether it be the maintenance of normal function or a response to a challenge aimed at restoring that normal function, all three of the considerations can be seen to be involved at some stage. Indeed, many of the physiological processes conventionally described in such detail can be seen to have components of each broad directing force within them. But their activities are *balanced and interrelated.* Normal life and health is dependent on the continuous and dynamic interaction between these three fundamental types of physiological process, resulting in the maintenance of a harmonious state. In a perfectly healthy individual the physiological forces will be in balance, and will always remain so. But it is a dynamic, constantly fluctuating balance, always adapting to meet the needs of the moment, then either returning to its previous equilibrium or creating a new balance dictated by new needs.

Thus any challenge will be met by a temporary increase in those physiological activities necessary to restore and maintain the integrity of the whole. This inevitably results for a time in an imbalance between the activities, with each taking place to the degree and in the order required by the situation being faced. But it is a controlled and temporary imbalance, which is corrected as soon as the challenge has been adequately dealt with. This concept of *fluctuating and dynamic balance* is essential for an understanding of the function of the body and the role of miasms in disturbing that function – and thus creating clinical disease. It is important to remember that under normal circumstances the balance is maintained not only within a particular body system, and between the processes taking place within that system, but also at the same time between different systems.

The Maintenance of Balance

The maintenance of this fluctuating balance is the means whereby the influence that Hahnemann described as the 'vital force' ensures what is now understood as homeostasis. He describes it in Paragraph 9 of the *Organon* as the force 'that enlivens the material organism as *dynamis*, governs without restriction and keeps all parts of the organism in admirable, harmonious, vital operation', and his footnote to Paragraph 22 describes the vital force as being 'only installed in our organism to continue our life on a harmonious course'. The processes themselves are not, of course, that force – they are only the channels through which it manifests. However, the need for balance is of a higher, non-material and more dynamic nature than just basic physiological homeostasis. It encompasses the emotional and mental aspects of being, and hence the balance is necessary at all levels and is self-regulating. It is perhaps not quite the vital force itself, lacking as it does any 'spiritual' or 'immaterial' element. But it is certainly an integral part of the concept.

The constant and appropriate adjustments to the body's balance that occur all the time are necessary for the maintenance of health. If, for any reason, a correct and appropriate response to challenge is not possible, illness and finally pathology will result. For as long as such unbalancing and obstructive influences persist, no response can be appropriate and correct. This is consistent with what Hahnemann meant when he said about chronic diseases in Paragraph 78 of the *Organon* that 'when left to themselves (without the use of remedies that are specific against them) these diseases go on increasing. Even with the best mental and bodily dietetic conduct, they mount until the end of life, … the best regulated lifestyle, and the most vigorous energy of the life force are not in a position to eradicate them.' The vital force maintains normal life through the fluctuating yet balanced functioning of the three fundamental activities discussed above. In the presence of a miasm, the vital force will be unable to overcome it, as the very means through which the vital force is attempting to work – that is, the ability to rebalance the body's functions – has been lost due to the presence of the miasm. The resulting enforced loss of balance is itself the root of the problem.

Physiologically, the three basic physical types of function may be summarised as 'production', 'removal' and 'regulation'. Because the physical and mental spheres are all part of the same whole, and governed by the same forces, each of these has a corresponding action and function on the higher planes, and all mental reactions can also be classified within one of the three types of function. Thus anger falls within the sphere of production, acceptance/forgiveness corresponds to removal, and calmly getting on with life is regulation. This is true of all species. Some modern interpretations of the miasms in fact concentrate more on their mental and emotional aspects than on their physical manifestations. Mentally these functions are manifest respectively as creativity, selectivity and perseverance.

Classifications of Body Functions

The three normal types of function and their variations as discussed above can form the basis of classifications of the dynamics of the body. Grauvogl (1811–1877) was a German homeopath who, in 1866, produced a classification of body types based on what he described as their 'biochemical state' (published in his *Textbook of Homoeopathy*, 1870). These states reflected the variations of symptoms that were observed, especially in relation to the reactions to climate. He identified three basic types, which he called the hydrogenoid, the oxygenoid and the carbonitrogenoid.

Although Hahnemann himself introduced the first thoughts about constitutional remedies, with his comments about Nitric Acid in *Chronic Diseases,* Grauvogl's approach broadened the concept of constitution towards how it is understood today, and he even went as far as ascribing certain remedies as being appropriate for the treatment of particular types. His classification was based on Hahnemann's ideas, although he interpreted the basic miasmatic concepts in relation to the chemical functioning of the body. However, there are similarities between the two approaches, as both are based on the functional reactions of the body and their variations in disease. The relationship between the two is discussed in the relevant chapters on the individual miasms.

Grauvogl's concept was later generally replaced by that of Nebel (1870–1954), a French homeopath who introduced the idea of typology into his classification. He too postulated three types, which he called the carbonic, fluoric and phosphoric. Although there are some overlaps between his ideas and those of Hahnemann and Grauvogl, the introduction of the morphological aspect moves him away from the purely functional considerations of the previous interpretations towards a system based on physical form, and this can lead to some confusion in relation to understanding the true nature of miasms. (Nebel also introduced a further complication by being one of the first to talk about a separate tubercular miasm in addition to the basic three that Hahnemann had described.)

The Origins of Miasms

Hahnemann's original miasms of sycosis, syphilis and psora can be considered as arising from the intrinsic functioning of the body in health and disease. The major miasmatic characteristics, as they are seen clinically, may be summarised as excess, destruction and deficiency. These broad characteristics, as with Grauvogl's types, can be considered as having their origins in the three normal types of function discussed above, namely production, removal and control.

Viewing the miasms as *functional entities* is one key to the understanding of chronic disease. Continuous and normal function is the essence of healthy life. Disease is produced by malfunction, and malfunction always precedes pathology. The primary physiological forces, and the miasms, represent three different ways in which the body functions, or malfunctions, in both health and disease. The themes of the miasms and their associated normal functions represent the normal progress of life. The terminology that homeopaths employ when talking about 'dis-ease' – as distinct from 'disease' – is particularly appropriate when considering the miasms. In a case of chronic disease the three processes are all still going on, as they would be in a perfectly healthy body. For reasons that are discussed later, they will each have become either under- or over-active, and it is the loss of balance (or ease) between them which produces the clinical picture of a miasm that is recognised.

Thus the process of regeneration and new growth, if taken to excess, becomes the sycotic miasm with its theme of *overproduction and overreaction.* The beneficial activity of the removal and elimination of obsolete material or dangerous agents develops pathologically into the *self-destruction and perversion* of the syphilitic influence. And the control and self-regulation of the whole, when distorted, manifests as psora in the form of either a frank *deficiency* or as a *failure to control* the internal environment and maintain homeostasis. This results in the failure of the self-regulatory mechanisms which provides a control of the other two activities. This inevitably leads to a loss of the essential balance, which itself may be regarded as a form of deficiency.

Chronic Disease

It is important to bear in mind the homeopathic concept of chronic disease as compared to the conventional interpretation. Conventionally, the criteria are primarily concerned with the presence of a particular pathology or malfunction in a particular system, together with its presence over a period of time. There is often also an implication, and acceptance, of incurability in the condition. Homeopathically, time is also an important factor, but in addition there is the realisation that the expression of chronic illness involves a deep-seated involvement of the whole body, with the particular signs and symptoms varying over time and often appearing in different systems of the body on different occasions. When it is realised that the true nature of chronic disease is an upset in the balance between the primary physiological forces of the body, then the inevitability of the widespread nature of the condition becomes apparent. All organs and tissues function within the constraints of these forces, and hence any deep imbalance is capable of producing manifestations anywhere in the body. Various factors, which are discussed later, determine the exact clinical picture in any particular case, but the potential for universal involvement is always there.

A Model of 'Dis-ease'

The author proposes a model which, although theoretical, provides a means of understanding the functioning of the body in disease. This envisages that a hypothetical perfectly balanced and healthy individual, under no challenge, can be represented as an equilateral triangle. Each side represents one of the three basic physiological functions, which between them cover the whole range of the processes necessary for life. By this definition the triangle will have all three sides of equal length. In the working of the model the shape of the triangle will change as described below and the length of the individual sides will vary, but the total length of the three sides will always remain the same. At this stage of the model the functions represented are all operating within normal limits:

Figure 1: *The body in perfect health*

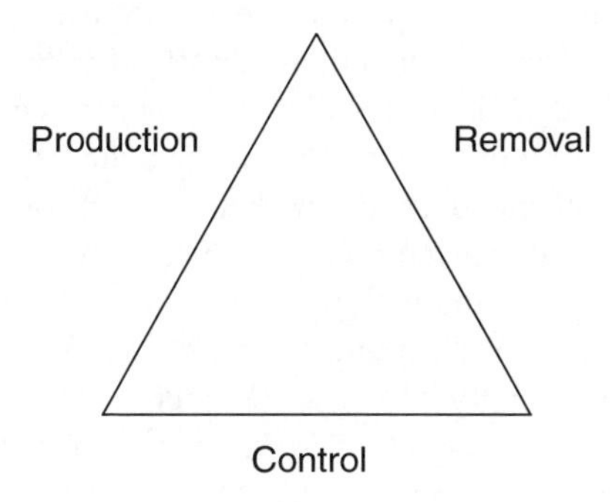

In the event of a challenge the balance will shift in such a way as to provide the necessary response to meet that particular challenge. For example, in the case of an infection, the temperature will become elevated and there will be the creation of more neutrophils and other leucocytes – the so-called shift to the left in the blood cell picture. This represents an increase in production. The resulting increased phagocytosis and destruction of the invading organisms is part of the removal function. In order for these functions to increase their activity as required by the situation, the control element in the balance must reduce (rather like letting a guard dog off the leash to deal with intruders). The resulting triangle may be represented as below, with an increase primarily in the production side, a lesser increase in the removal arm and a corresponding reduction in the control wing:

Figure 2: *The body under acute challenge*

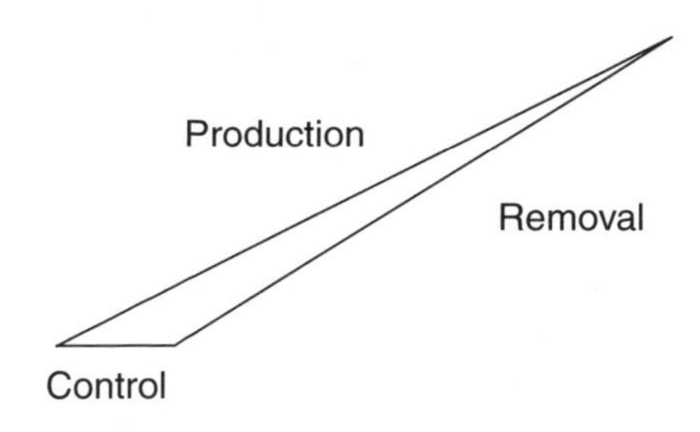

Deviation from the equilateral nature of the triangle is inevitable in any response situation, but a balance between the functions must be maintained to preserve any semblance of normality, and within the concept of this model it is essential for life that the integrity of the triangle is preserved. This means that, as shown above, any increase in the activity of one or more functions must be matched by changes in the activities of the others to accommodate it. It is of course possible, indeed common, that the required response to a particular challenge involves an increase in the activity of two of the functions. If this is the case then the model will require that the activity of the third function must correspondingly decrease in order to accommodate this. In Figure 2 (page 19) the reduction in the control function represents a loosening of the restraints on the other two functions that enables them to respond to the challenge in an appropriate manner.

In an acute case, once the infection has been overcome, the situation represented in Figure 2 will theoretically revert to that of Figure 1, i.e. a state of homeostasis, by means of a re-establishment of the control function. But because the normal state of health is a constantly fluctuating balance this does not occur. In practice what will happen is that a new challenge will result in a new temporary imbalance to meet the changing situation. But the aim, even though it is generally unobtainable due to constant new challenges, *will always be to return to the situation of perfect balance represented by Figure 1,* as this represents the condition of perfect health. And it is important to realise that in this hypothetical example there is no *intrinsic* reason why the perfect balance cannot be re-established. It is only external factors that will prevent it.

It is also important to realise that all physiological reactions in the body involve elements of all three types of function, and hence, as is discussed below, all disease situations contain elements of all three processes.

In chronic disease the situation is rather different. Here the balance represented in Figure 2 has not returned to the position shown in Figure 1 after an acute challenge, but has itself become the new balance that the body is seeking to return to. There is thus an adaptation to circumstances which appears to represent normality. Why this happens is discussed in the next chapter. But this new balance, *which is in fact abnormal* and is hence *dis-ease*, will govern all subsequent functioning of the body in both health and disease. If the preponderance of one type of function over the others in the new balance becomes great enough, then this will show either as a clinical entity or as a pattern running through a case. This is what is described as a miasmatic trait in the patient.

The Multimiasmatic Nature of Disease

Even if there is a strong presenting picture of one miasm in a disease situation, it must always be remembered that the other two activities are still there and functioning to some degree. In some cases these activities will remain within normal limits, but in others they too may be clinically miasmatic. They are capable of producing signs and symptoms even in the initial presentation of a case, when there is a predominant influence from one of the other forces: following treatment there may well be a change in the functional balance and their contribution to the overall picture may increase. Thus a case presenting primarily as colitis, with frequency and mucus in the stool, is predominantly an excess of both function and production, and is therefore sycotic. Another, but lesser, feature of the case may be a non-specific skin irritation, which will be psoric in origin. Following correct treatment, the colitis syndrome will ease and the skin symptoms may temporarily increase (this is also, of course, in accordance with Hering's Law).

As has been shown above, the model implies that *in every situation in both health and disease, all three functions and/or miasms are always there to some extent.* Within the model it is possible to have one function continuing to work normally, and hence its side of the triangle retains its original length, with the adjustments taking place in the other two sides in order to maintain the integrity of the whole. It should always be borne in the prescriber's mind that descriptions of a 'psoric', 'sycotic', or 'syphilitic' disease need to have the caveat *predominantly* applied to them. Accurate observation will always indicate that the other functions are also present to some degree. Depending on the individual case, there may have been sufficient disturbance to the body for those other functions to have acquired the status of a miasm rather than being seen as a physiologically normal form. This is important in relation to the 'newer' miasms and is discussed in more depth in Chapter 4.

It must always be remembered that normal function and miasmatic influences can exist together. Indeed, it is necessary for life that all three basic types of function continue to operate together. A miasmatic influence will inevitably overshadow a normal function (that is the nature of the miasm) but the normal function does not cease – it only changes.

Confusion can occur over the miasms when the same conventionally named clinical condition is attributed to different miasmatic influences in different individuals. The key to understanding this lies in realising, as stated above, that all situations contain elements of all three influences, and also that the functioning of all systems and organs is regulated by the balance between them in any particular case. What is important at all times is the balance of the physiological/miasmatic functions. If that balance becomes upset beyond a certain point in any direction, then the normal interaction of physiological function will fail. A recognised clinical condition is then seen, but the imbalance that produces it may be due to different influences in individual cases. Thus a case of colitis may present with spasm, abdominal pain and explosive diarrhoea, which will be associated with a sycotic influence. However, another case, also classed as colitis, may show ulceration, bleeding and symptoms associated more with the destructive nature of the syphilitic miasm. The former will be described as sycotic in origin, whereas the latter would be described as syphilitic. Yet in the latter case there is still a significant sycotic element. The difference lies in the greater degree of the syphilitic miasm present in the case, which changes the detailed symptomatology. Similarly, appendicitis is basically sycotic, and a typical acute case would be classified as such. However, a 'grumbling appendix' with indistinct symptoms could be classed as psoric due to the influence of psora, and an infected case with rupture and peritonitis would be manifesting a significant syphilitic element.

The Multimiasmatic Nature of the Patient

Every individual is born with an accumulation of miasmatic 'baggage', the exact nature of which depends on inherited factors. This will subsequently be added to and altered as a result of the person's or animal's experiences and challenges. Correct homeopathic treatment and disease management in the early stages of life can reduce the imbalances, but in many cases the result of exposure to challenge is a reinforcement of the miasms already present and hence of the unbalanced state.

The concept of the possibility of the constitutional remedy of an individual changing through life is widely accepted, and in those cases where the remedy does not change, this is taken as evidence of a strong constitution. Another view, based on clinical experience (Beattie, 1999; Armstrong, 2003) is that there is a triad of remedies which together make up the constitutional picture of a patient rather than one single remedy,. These three can be regarded as reflecting the underlying miasmatic makeup in that particular individual. Which one is required as treatment at any particular time will depend on the exact circumstances of the patient, together with the exact nature of the challenge. Over time it will be found in many cases that there is a pattern of prescribing around the same three remedies, and that this represents the fluctuations in the inbuilt miasmatic patterns of that body in response to life's requirements. However, it also always represents an *imbalance* in the physiological functioning of the patient.

The Effects of Treatment

Following successful homeopathic treatment with a well-selected remedy there will be a reduction in the predominant activity of the major miasm in the case. This will allow either another, previously secondary, miasmatic influence to exert itself, thereby producing a new set of symptoms, or the normal physiological activity of one or both of the other influences to be resumed to a greater or lesser degree. Further correct treatment selected on the new presenting picture will repeat the process, until in theory the perfect equilibrium is once more established.

In the very early stages of a chronic disease there may be a similarity to such an over-simple scenario. But in most cases the situation will be much more complicated, with the three functions being greatly intertwined and complicating each other. But nevertheless the above is essentially the process of the cure in all cases of chronic disease. This is often described as dealing with the situation layer by layer. When a point in a case is reached when the normal physiological processes can once more function in balance, then cure is possible.

Within the triangular model, the presence of a strong sycotic and/ or syphilitic miasm – as is found in many cases of longstanding chronic disease – implies, in order to maintain the triangle, that there will be an inevitable reduction in normal control activity. (This must, however, not be confused with the deficiency of the true psoric miasm. It is a secondary rather than a primary reduction, and represents a normal adjustment on the part of the body rather than further miasmatic activity.) As long as this situation continues the disease process will remain essentially internalised. As the two miasms are contained or eliminated as a result of treatment, the normal control activity will increase. It will be seen in Chapter 5 that the appearance of lesions on the skin does not invariably indicate a psoric *miasm,* but may in fact indicate a restoration of normal function, thus enabling the body to throw the disease outwards in accordance with Hering's Law.

Hahnemann said in *Chronic Diseases* that the final stage in the successful treatment of any chronic disease is the reappearance of the psoric miasm. In fact it is likely that it is the restoration of normal control function that results in Hering's Law being able once more to operate, producing the external appearance of the disease process as the final stage. Hence, ulceration appearing on the skin following treatment may be a combination of Hering's Law working on a syphilitic influence.

Chapter 3

The Basic Miasms as Clinical Entities

The Immune System as a Functional Entity

Conventionally, the immune system is regarded as the means whereby the body guards against and eliminates illness. But the full immune *function* of the body involves much more than just the activities of one conventionally defined body system. It is concerned not only with the defence against external challenge but also with the maintenance of the whole normal internal environment of the body, and it is because of this that there is the close involvement and interaction of a number of systems, notably the immune and the endocrine.

Although, as has already been discussed, all three basic types of function, i.e. production, removal and control, are always present in every situation, it is nevertheless possible to recognise a predominant tendency towards certain of these basic functions in particular systems, linked to the overriding physiological requirements of that system's function. It must be emphasised that not only are the functions themselves physiological here – as opposed to pathological and therefore miasmatic – but that the bias towards particular functions within a system is also purely physiological. There is no suggestion of miasmatic, and therefore abnormal, predominance in these normal situations. Thus, because the endocrine system is primarily concerned with the maintenance of the internal environment of the body, the emphasis within that system is towards a state of control, and the tendency towards a state of miasmatic psora within the system is, in many cases, the natural development in chronic disease.

Similarly, because the immune function as a whole is as much concerned with maintaining the status quo as with repelling challenges, the former function means that the system may be tipped easily into a psoric state. However, because the normal balance of the physiological functions within the immune system is fairly equal, a more sycotic and/or syphilitic picture often develops as a consequence of the requirements of meeting acute challenges, with the inevitable upset to the regulatory control that is involved. The exact picture that emerges will depend very much on the nature of the challenge that triggered it.

While this is not an absolute rule, it is valuable as a general guide, although the possibility of one or both of the other basic miasms manifesting within any system must always be borne in mind. This is where the interrelationship of function between systems comes into play. It is interesting to note that sycotic activity is often seen in the endocrine glands most closely linked to the immune system, such as the thyroid.

But it is primarily through the activities and abuses of the immune response that miasmatic states become established, and it is these mechanisms that must now be examined.

The Creation of Miasms

One integral part of the functioning of the immune response is the process and direction of cure as outlined by Hering's Law. The working through of this process is important for the restoration of balance between the physiological functions once the need for a response to challenge has been met. As has been shown, the original hypothetical perfection is never immediately recreated, but the new balances that are created, as the response proceeds, should be governed by the natural direction of cure. If the working through of Hering's Law is blocked, then the process is forced back upon itself. For as long as the block remains, an abnormal relationship between the primary physiological forces will be present. The body will adjust these to create what balance it can, but it will inevitably be an abnormal balance that will then become the new norm. This leads to a situation where the body can neither develop its responses to their full extent nor return to the normal perfect state. Thus suppression of disease can in itself lead to the creation of a miasmatic state.

Throughout all his writings on the subject Hahnemann stressed the role of suppression in the creation of miasms as clinical entities. In *Chronic Diseases* he constantly emphasises the necessity of not just treating the external signs of disease, and instances the subsequent development of the internal miasmatic disease when this is done, at one point citing ninety-seven cases in support of his contention. In the footnote to Paragraph 205 of the *Organon*, he draws attention to the adverse consequences following the removal of facial and breast cancers without addressing the underlying disease. Nor was he alone in these observations. He quotes with approval the writing of L.C. Juncker who describes cases of piles, catarrh, colic and renal gravel arising as a result of the suppression of skin symptoms (*Dissertatio de Damno ex Scabie Repulsa*, 1750). In his *Instructions for Surgeons Respecting Venereal Diseases* (1798) he quotes John Hunter (1728–1793), the father of British surgery: 'The result of destroying the chancre ever so early … if this is effected by local applications, was always the consequent outbreak of syphilis': and also 'not one patient out of fifteen will escape syphilis if the chancre is destroyed by mere external applications'. Later J.H. Allen, in *The Chronic Miasms*, gives numerous case histories in support of Hahnemann's interpretation.

It has been postulated (Miles, 1992; Norland, 2003) that allowing the young to experience and overcome non-life-threatening disease as part of the maturing process can help in the clearing from the body of any miasmic influences that may have been inherited. Recently (Adler, 2005) a review of epidemiological evidence has queried this. However this review was concerned only with atopy in relation to the 'hygiene hypothesis' of allergy causation. Experience has shown that overzealous prevention of these diseases may not be in the best interests of the developing body. The same argument can apply to the overuse of antibiotics and other agents to combat acute disease in the young (which conclusion is supported by Adler's review). Too vigorous a use of these can abort the working-through of the disease process, and hence create a suppression.

In the animal world the use of vaccines against kennel cough in dogs and chlamydia in cats, both of which are non-life-threatening conditions, may be counterproductive, and in the human field some of the childhood diseases may well come into the same category. This idea fits in with the above concept, as the body is allowed to follow its natural processes without undue interference to their natural conclusion. Indeed, any working of the immune system – even at a minimal clinical level, when an infection is overcome with only mild symptoms developing – which is allowed to proceed without interruption is potentially beneficial. The use of homeopathic remedies such as Sulphur, Calcarea Carbonica and Tuberculinum, all in the 200c potency, in the role of eugenic agents to assist the developing foetal system to cope with and adjust its miasmatic inheritance has been advocated in this regard (Day, 1984; Wolff, 1984), and to this end various regimes administered via the mother during pregnancy have been employed. A commonly advocated regime is a single dose of each remedy, in the above order, at three-day intervals as early in pregnancy as possible.

Against that, Elmiger (1998) has opposed the practice, arguing that treatment of both parents prior to conception is the only effective means of countering miasmatic influences. The author's experience would support the concept of foetal treatment.

In the absence of any such precautionary treatment, further suppression of diseases, either by treatment or vaccination, can result in the reinforcing of the inherited miasms. A similar situation can arise when the suppression is not of an immune response related to disease but of another normal physiological process connected with other aspects of life, e.g. reproduction. In these cases the relevant systems, although capable of reacting normally, are not being allowed to do so. But the normal processes will not cease to try to function as nature intended. The result of this is that if the normal outcome of the process is blocked, then another outcome will be established. If the abuse of suppression continues for too long this may ultimately result in the establishment of a miasmatic imbalance within the system. This can then lead to the appearance of pathology created by the dominant miasm.

Equally serious consequences can arise where the immune system has been conditioned to react abnormally. There are two ways in which this can happen.

Firstly, if there is exposure to a too severe challenge at an early stage of development, then the functional integrity of the immune response may be compromised. The newborn immune system, as with the rest of the body, requires time to mature, and although, of necessity, it matures more quickly than many of the other systems, that does not change its basic requirement. Maturity implies balance and a measured response to any given situation, and balance, as has been shown, is the prerequisite of normal health. Immaturity has a potential for imbalance, and a consequent inability to function to best advantage.

Nature goes to great lengths to protect the immature immune system, such as the provision of maternal antibodies to prevent not only the death of the young, but, perhaps more importantly, to prevent the young system from having to cope with a challenge that it is unprepared for. However, when there is a breakdown of that protection, such as when it is overridden by early vaccination, then potentially there is an excessive and inappropriate response to challenge – high fever for no necessary reason, etc. This can occur as an isolated incident with no long-term consequences, but if the breakdown occurs due to the intrinsically virulent nature of the challenge and/or the overriding of parts of the normal defence process, then more permanent imbalances can be created, which show as miasms. Abuse of the vaccination procedure can lead to the creation of a sycotic state (Burnett, 1897; Fortier-Bernovillie, 1934). In practice the immature body that receives the challenge will be carrying some inherited miasmatic influences already, just as it will have inherited other characteristics from its parents, and these new shocks to the system will reinforce or alter that existing imbalance.

The second situation is when the immune system is subjected to repeated challenges from the same agent, which will stimulate the same balance of response every time. The miasmatic nature of disease agents is discussed below, but if a system is conditioned by experience to react to a particular challenge in the same way time and time again, it finally becomes conditioned to react to all challenges in that particular way. Regular exposure over a period of time to highly virulent infections requiring a marked rise in temperature as a necessary part of the body's response may result in a situation where the body will respond with a high temperature to any challenge, even if it is of a non-infectious nature. Once firmly established, this conditioning may be passed to subsequent generations. If the initial repeated exposures are to an immature system the results will be even more marked. These effects may be part of the story in the creation of the tubercular miasm.

The Inheritance of Miasms

In the footnote to Paragraph 282 of the *Organon*, Hahnemann writes that 'Psora is usually communicated through breast milk to most nursing infants, if they do not already possess it by inheritance from the mother.' Burnett (1897) considered that vaccinosis could be transmitted in the same way. In the author's view, vaccinosis is not itself a miasm, but rather a chronic disease state induced as a result of vaccination, with its exact manifestation being based on miasms. Hence the observed clinical fact of its transmission is some evidence for the inheritance of miasms. In the present day, with the widespread use of vaccination, inherited miasmatic influences as a result of the practice will inevitably add to the problems arising as a consequence of vaccination in the young. In addition, there is no doubt, from what is observed in clinical practice, that miasmic influences can be inherited in some way. The trail of previous family illness that practitioners look for as part of their case-taking is a reflection of this. The presence of allergic or neoplastic traits in families is often linked to the miasmatic pattern that is passed through the generations, as is the widespread presence of what is recognised as the tubercular miasm in cattle, in spite of the fact that for many years there was a relatively low incidence of the clinical disease. J.H. Allen, in *The Chronic Miasms* states in relation to the tubercular miasm that miasms are 'perfectly combined by hereditary transmission'.

The mechanism for the inheritance of miasms is not entirely clear, although various possibilities have been suggested. Certain inherited conditions show definite miasmatic connections, but the concept cannot be related to a clear-cut inheritance in the conventional genetic sense in every case. Changes in the makeup of the DNA as a result of previous miasmatic activity have been postulated as a possible route (Elliott, 1996). Another view is that the DNA complex is in effect an electromagnetic transmitter/receiver, and that it is through this mechanism that the changes occur, with the patterns of balance (or imbalance) being held as energy imprints within the complex (Rost and Rost, 1986). However, since what is being considered here are basic forces directing the conventional biological processes of the body, it is perhaps more appropriate to regard them rather in the same way as the vital force is viewed, as higher dynamic forces rather than physical entities.

In the modern world it is inevitable that every living body is born with a certain amount of inherited vulnerability due to miasmatic influences. Vaccination, as mentioned above, is one source. The suppressive nature of much orthodox treatment can also have an effect on subsequent generations, as witnessed by the alarming increase in allergic conditions in recent times (see Chapter 7). Mention has been made above of the possible role of early illness in clearing this. If there is no such cleansing experience then, as has been discussed, the congenital miasmatic pattern will remain and be built on, potentially adding further instability to an already unstable situation. If such early illness can clear the miasmatic influences, then the individual will be able to respond to future challenges in a more balanced way. As would be expected, the more firmly entrenched a miasmatic pattern is, the more difficult it is to clear.

It is thus that miasms give the greatest predisposition to disease, which is what is meant by *diathesis*. This is not quite the same thing as a straightforward miasmatic influence, although the two terms are often considered to be interchangeable (see below). The presence of any miasms will influence the way that a body responds to whatever challenge comes its way, but as long as the response can incorporate the facility for a fluctuating balance (see Chapter 2), there is the possibility that this can be dealt with. The less flexibility there is in the situation, as is discussed in Chapter 4, the more the body is hampered in its efforts to defend itself, and the more susceptible it is to challenge. Also, the less the natural responses are allowed to function, the more erratic and / or exaggerated the response is likely to be.

Diathesis and Constitution

There is much confusion surrounding these terms, with different interpretations being placed on each, and with an overlap between those interpretations. Diathesis has been defined as either 'A pattern of disorder characteristic of an underlying disease trait' (*International Dictionary of Homeopathy*, 2000) or as 'The inherited or acquired organic weakness and systemic inferiority which leads to the morbid dispositions and specific pathological processes in the evolution of a disease' (Koehler, 1986). It may thus be regarded as predisposition to a particular named disease. This, of course, implies a particular pre-set miasmatic pattern. On the other hand, a clear clinical miasm is a predisposition to particular types of reactions following disease challenges in general. The sensitivity of particular individuals to certain remedies may be connected to their miasmatic makeup. Similarly the constitutional type and miasmatic type have many overlaps, but they are not quite the same thing. The constitutional type – which is essentially the mental and physical characteristics and reactions of the individual in the healthy state – will be greatly affected by the inherited miasmatic make-up of that individual but will also contain elements over and above that, as other elements of heredity will ensure a broader picture. In contrast, the miasmatic picture on its own becomes of major clinical importance in the disease state.

Acute and Latent Miasms

These terms, which are often used in connection to miasms, can also be confusing. The terminology 'an acute miasm' can be especially so, even though Hahnemann uses it on several occasions in both the *Organon* and *Chronic Diseases*. He used the term to separate what he called 'the more superficial diseases', essentially what are now recognised as the infectious and epidemic diseases, from the genuine deep-seated chronic diseases. Kent, in his *Lectures on Homoeopathic Philosophy* (XVIII) draws a clear distinction between acute and chronic miasms. To understand the difference, it is necessary to discard the orthodox definition of chronic as being based solely on time. From the homeopathic point of view it is the intrinsic nature of the condition that makes it chronic, not the length of time it has been present. Kent states: 'A chronic miasm is chronic from its beginning, and an acute miasm is acute from its beginning.' Koehler (1986) defines the essential difference as 'Whether the organism is able to overcome the illness by itself or medical treatment is necessary to achieve this end' (by medical treatment he means prolonged homeopathic treatment). Banerjee (1931) states that it is the inherent nature of the disease that makes it either acute or chronic. Thus, as the term is often currently used, it is really a misnomer, as the essence of the miasmatic concept centres around the reactions of the body in chronic disease. One modern concept of the acute miasm is an extension of a view of miasms that links them intrinsically to various life stages, and stages of a disease process, essentially irrespective of particular diseases (Sankaran, 1994). As its name suggests, it is essentially an acute response to sudden challenge, and this was the sense in which both Hahnemann and Kent used it. It must, of course, by definition, include all the three primary physiological functions of production, removal and control in the reaction.

In *Chronic Diseases*, Hahnemann also mentions 'half-acute' miasms, and cites rabies as an example of an infection producing no eruption. However, it appears to the author that there is considerable doubt over this concept, as Hahnemann bases his interpretation on observations that appear to take no account of any differential diagnosis of aggression in dogs. Although in his 'Thoughts suggested by the recommendation of a remedy for the effects of the bite of mad dogs' (*Lesser Writings*, 1803; Dudgeon's translation, 1853) he addresses this issue to some extent, he still maintains his position as set out in *Chronic Diseases*. He states that in his experience only 'one out of twenty or thirty who are bitten' become infected. Even the experience that he quotes of others that one in twelve succumb is so far at odds with modern experience as to demand some explanation. The virulent nature of the true rabies virus must be a significant factor.

A latent miasm has a validity within the traditional theory. Hahnemann attributed many acute fevers to the presence of latent psora (*Organon*, Paragraph 73). The predisposition in a body to a particular type of reaction in the face of challenge can result in the presence, and subsequent manifestation, of latent miasms. Since, from the homeopathic perspective, all disease is a dynamic disturbance at an energetic level, latent miasms may be thought of as energy patterns of previous experiences and response patterns that are still in the body, but it must be remembered that the original illness may have been in a previous generation. In a perfect world the acute response to challenge would involve the model as described in Figure 1 of Chapter 2. What occurs in reality is that the body does not start its response from the state represented in Figure 1 but from that in Figure 2, which is already in a state of imbalance. If that imbalance is great enough, then it will already be showing clinically as a miasm, with the exact symptom picture being dependent on the prominent influence.

Thus a psoric pattern may show as a case of psoriasis, a sycotic as chronic cystitis or a syphilitic as an ulcerative condition. If it is much milder there may well be the appearance of something approaching normality in spite of its presence, and a patient, when asked, may state that they are well. Owners may claim that their animals are healthy. However, the imbalance will still be there and if the vital force is disturbed sufficiently, once the acute phase is over, the initial imbalance will be reinforced and show as a clinical entity. If the miasmatic tendency of the challenge, and discussed in Chapter 6, is similar to the latent miasm, the resulting clinical picture will be correspondingly severe. If its balance is different then the final outcome will be milder, but the latent miasm can still have become active. The uncorrected course of many chronic diseases will show variation between periods of frank miasmatic activity and more quiescent, latent intervals, but in many of these cases there will be slight signs of a lurking influence waiting to flare.

System Affinities of the Miasms

Miasms can be regarded as essentially unbalanced functional entities that have their origins in the normal functional activities of the body. They arise when these functions are not allowed to operate in the way nature intended, due to the inappropriate suppression of either disease response or normal physiological function. In a normal body, different systems have different priorities of function in the broader scheme of life and survival, and these functions will require different balances of the basic physiological forces in order to fulfil their roles. Individual cells and tissues within a system may have their own different functional role, but nevertheless there can be seen in particular systems a tendency towards certain activities that are of particular value to the organism as a whole.

The general role of the endocrine system in the maintenance of the internal environment of the body has been mentioned. The nervous system, via its autonomic component, is also closely involved with the maintenance of normality and a balanced function. The reproductive system has a strongly physiological leaning towards the creation of new tissue. A similar functional imperative can be seen in the need for the removal of foreign matter and invaders via the immune system. These become of great importance when there is suppression of normal function for whatever reason, and in these circumstances there may well be a conversion from physiological to miasmatic activity. This occurs because the importance of the physiological function to the organism as a whole means that the body will endeavour to maintain that function, even against the suppression. The result of this is often that a system with a strong natural functional priority will ultimately, rather than cease the function, turn that function in on itself and produce pathology. It is largely because of this distribution of function within the body that the known clinical expressions of suppressed miasmatic activity are seen. There is a tendency for suppression to create a miasm in those systems and tissues most predisposed towards its normal functional equivalent. This is discussed in later chapters as appropriate, but is why underactivity of endocrine glands is seen as a result of psora, uterine growths arise from sycosis and autoimmune disease has a strong syphilitic component.

Natural Outlets for Miasms

The bias that certain systems have towards particular physiological activities has implications for the treatment of miasmatic disease. The body will naturally attempt to use these systems as an outlet for, and means of clearing, existing miasms that have an affinity with the particular systems: successful homeopathic treatment will, by its very nature, encourage this process. The body's chosen route of response will always be towards exteriorising as far as possible the manifestations of disease and maximising the effectiveness of healing (Paragraph 201 of the *Organon* should be read in its entirety, together with Hering's Law). If these outlets are blocked, then the potential effect is to drive the chronic disease deeper into the body, and hence to accentuate the malfunction, with a resulting increase in pathology and slow but steady deterioration of the patient's general health. As will be seen in Chapter 5, as well as the disease process going deeper into the more vital organs, the miasmatic effects tend to increase in severity, with the sycotic and then the syphilitic activities becoming more prominent. This does not mean that the body will only use such outlets, but they are major 'safety valves' and their blocking can lead to increased activity in other directions. For example, the complete removal of the uterus and ovaries can result in pathology appearing in the mammary glands, those being the only remaining parts of the reproductive system, or the effects may be transferred to other systems, such as the respiratory with an increase in catarrhal discharges from the nasal mucosa, the urinary with chronic cystitis, or the muscular with a marked increase in cramps and pains. In individual cases the body may be able to compensate for such a loss of a major outlet by finding another on the surface of the body, but in others it will merely result in a deepening of the chronic disease pattern.

Hahnemann defined the main natural outlet for psora as via the mucous and cutaneous surfaces of the body, the most common result being pruritis. This has been confirmed by the observations of many practitioners, with the addition of the appearance of diarrhoea – in spite of the fact that the normal/latent state for psora is towards constipation, as the lining of the bowel is continuous with the skin and hence the two will often act together – with the possibility of untoward consequences resulting from the artificial removal of these symptoms. Sycosis finds its main release via the urogenital system, and the possible consequences of interfering with this are discussed in detail in Chapter 4. Case 1 (page 59) at the end of that chapter shows the possible ramifications of the phenomenon. The syphilitic miasm is the one that has the least system affinity in this context, although there is some affinity with the reproductive system. In addition, the body's aim generally with syphilis is one of exteriorisation via ulceration.

Basic Forces in Nature

The three primary functional forces of production, removal and control that are seen in the body as physiological processes are mirrored in other aspects of nature. The first of these situations is in the remedies themselves. Remedies are essentially functional entities and each remedy will exhibit elements of all the three functions that are seen in the body. The proportions will vary with each remedy *but always be unique and constant.* Thus, as in Chapter 2, where disease was designated as predominantly of one miasmatic type or another, so appropriate remedies should always be thought of as *predominantly* showing the pattern of one particular miasm while still retaining aspects of the other two influences. And while remedies are commonly spoken of as being psoric, sycotic or syphilitic, it must be remembered that they are in fact *anti*, as the aim and effect of treatment is to cure. Thus, for example, an accurate description of Thuja should be 'a predominantly antisycotic remedy', whereas in everyday clinical conversation it is usually referred to as a 'sycotic remedy'.

In the model outlined in Chapter 2 Thuja would thus be represented as:

Figure 3: *Antimiasmatic representation of Thuja*

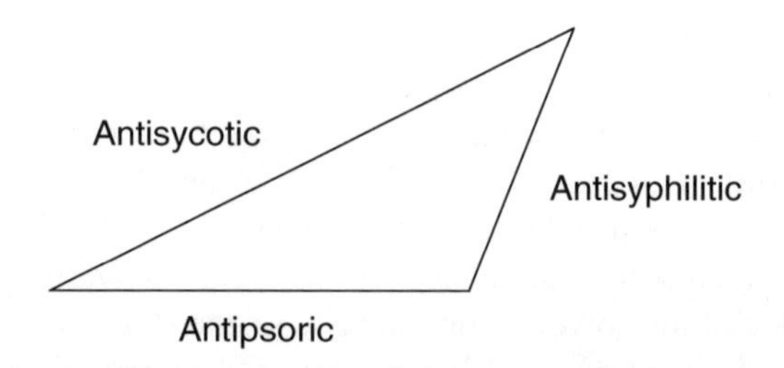

The antisycotic side of the triangle is extended as a reflection of the predominantly antisycotic nature of the remedy. This extension is largely at the expense of the antisyphilitic activity, while the antipsoric element is still present to a significant degree. If the materia medica of Thuja is compared with the model as above, it will be seen that the majority of the symptoms described, such as warts, pigmentation, chronic catarrh, hurried behaviour, balanitis, aggravation in damp weather and many others, plus the major sites of action being the skin and urogenital organs, are all attributable to the sycotic influence. Similarly dry eruptions, dirty-looking skin, impotence, weakness in limbs and others are a reflection of psora. Few syphilitic symptoms are found, being limited to some bone pains around the face and teeth, painful ulcers around the mouth and the production of foul and infected pustules on the skin.

In contrast, Calcarea Carbonica, which, with its theme of imperfect nutrition, general weakness and inactivity is generally considered to be a major antipsoric remedy, and was described by Hahnemann as such, can be regarded as having a considerable antisycotic component, and significant aspects of its remedy picture, such as the warts and exostoses, renal colic with calculi and cramps in limbs, point to this latter miasm.

Figure 4: *Antimiasmatic representation of Calcarea Carbonica*

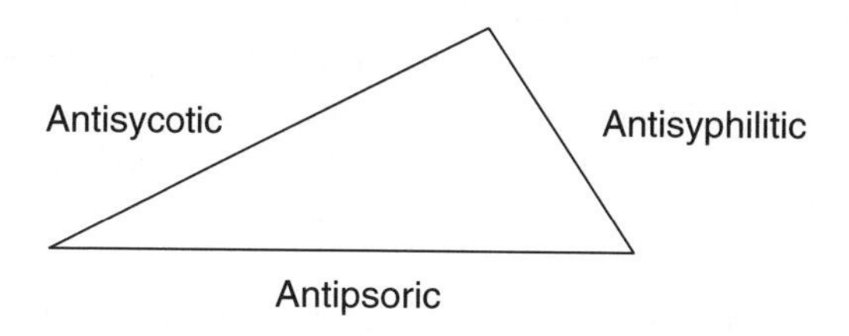

Although the warts seen in Thuja and Calcarea Carbonica are physically different, with those of Thuja being pedunculated (the more typical 'figwart'), whilst those of Calcarea are flatter, both are nevertheless a result of the sycotic influence.

Since what is being represented here is the *anti*miasmatic nature of the remedy, the diagrams above are in fact mirror-images of the type shown in Chapter 2, where what is being represented is miasmatic activity. The more closely the representations of the clinical picture and the remedy reflect each other, the nearer the treatment is to the simillimum. The reader is referred to Case 8 in Chapter 8 (page 109).

In many of the standard materia medica works, remedies are often described as only having one or two miasmatic connections. These may be the predominant ones, but it must be remembered that *all three functional connections are always there.* As indicated above, study of the materia medica of any well proven remedy will reveal individual symptoms that can be recognised as belonging to particular miasms, and inevitably all three types will be there to some degree.

Individual diseases and challenges also reflect an intrinsic miasmatic balance, and each will have its own components of deficiency, excess, and destruction, with the capacity to provoke the corresponding reaction in the body. Thus, for example, a predominantly sycotic challenge will provoke a predominantly sycotic response. The effect is an integral part of the cause, and *vice versa*. It is because of this that widespread individual diseases, such as tuberculosis, can lead to the establishment of miasmatic influences across whole generations and species. The continuous exposure of a population to the same challenge will generate a common response, and the miasmatic pattern of the disease thus established will imprint itself into the population's make-up due to the repeated exposure. As discussed above, this pattern can be passed down through the generations, perhaps being reinforced at each stage. The miasmatic pattern thus established can bring in its wake susceptibilities to a range of other diseases which share aspects of that pattern (Vithoulkas, 1980). This question of the miasmatic nature of particular challenges in relation to the selection of appropriate remedies is discussed further in Chapter 6. For the present it is sufficient to be aware that the basic forces which find expression physiologically in the normal processes of the body, and clinically in the miasms, are mirrored in the fundamental influences that are found throughout the whole of nature. And in general terms, the more virulent the challenge the more active will be the resulting influence of the sycotic and/or syphilitic miasms. Milder challenges, which produce only functional disturbances without physical damage, are reflected in a psoric response.

Miasmatic Tendencies within the Kingdoms

Because of the mirroring of nature's fundamental forces mentioned above, it is to be expected that the different kingdoms of the natural world would show different tendencies towards particular miasmatic influences, although these must not be regarded as absolute. As with remedies, all three influences can be seen to some degree in each kingdom. The plant kingdom tends towards the psoric, with some sycotic influences. This is in line with the concept of 'struggle' that is often associated with a psoric function. The speeding up and slowing down of the growth cycles that are seen in plants in accordance with the seasons mirrors the control of psora, and also the sycotic function, in the miasmatic influence.

The animal world has perhaps the greatest variety of miasmatic influences in the remedies it yields, but overall shows a tendency towards sycosis and syphilis. This is not surprising when the importance of the survival of the species is considered, given the very different requirements of animals as compared with plants. For an animal, strength and health equate with survival, and hence there is the instinct to both cover up weakness and to appear as big and strong as possible, in order to ensure that survival. Hiding and camouflage are also animal features, and all these represent a sycotic type of behaviour. The 'kill or be killed' nature of many species is mirrored in a syphilitic tendency. The mineral kingdom has leanings towards syphilis and psora. Minerals play a vital role in the daily metabolism of the body, which via homeostasis is connected to psora. The substantial nature of many minerals is concerned with structure and the maintenance of form. Failure of either of these leads on to the decay and destruction that is seen in the syphilitic miasm, which is such a strong feature of many mineral remedies.

In general terms, the position of an element in the periodic table, which is determined by its atomic weight, gives a broad indication of its miasmatic bias. Those at the upper end, having low weights, lean more towards the psoric influence, and the table leads through sycosis to the strongly syphilitic nature of the heavy metals with their high weights. In general terms the syphilitic tendency increases both from top to bottom and from left to right of the table.

The top two places in the table are occupied by hydrogen and helium, closely followed by elements such as carbon, oxygen and nitrogen, which were an integral part of the process by which life developed, and which are essential for its continuation. From the concept of psora as being involved in the struggles of life (Sankaran, 1994), remedies containing these elements would be expected to have strong antipsoric properties, and so it has proved. Such remedies are also among the most deep-acting in the materia medica (Sherr, 1992). Slightly below in the table are other elements vitally involved in the life process, among them being sodium, potassium, magnesium, iron and zinc. With these too there is a significant psoric influence, although a sycotic aspect is beginning to appear. Moving further down the table a syphilitic dimension begins to be seen, mainly at the expense of the psoric, until at the bottom are found the most strongly syphilitic elements such as lead, mercury and platinum. Since remedies are composed of the elements of the table in various combinations, the particular characteristics of those remedies will inevitably have a tendency to reflect the particular miasmatic traits and balances of the constituents.

Scholten's (1996) analysis of the periodic table and his concept of the elements, with the themes that he ascribes to his stages and series within the table, also reflect this changing pattern of the miasmatic influences. The elements, of course, form the basis for the structure and functioning of the bodies of all living things. Those that are not regularly used in the biochemical processes of life tend to be, intrinsically, the most destructive. Gold and platinum, whilst having no known physiological function in the body, are among the most strongly syphilitic of remedies, and at the extreme are the radioactive elements.

The concept of a universal kingdom has been suggested (Robbins, 2004), into which would fall such forces as sunlight, magnetism, fire and anti-matter – i.e. the energy forces – and hence the remedies derived from them. It would thus also include DNA and RNA, on the basis that everything in this kingdom is concerned with the major issues of creation and contains everything in an 'undifferentiated state'. By definition, such a kingdom would have all three of the basic forces strongly represented, with no overriding theme.

This concept is a development from the ideas of Rosenthal (2000), who has postulated an approach to homeopathy based on four kingdoms, designated as 'inanimate', 'plant', 'animal' and 'human', and their influence on the particular pathology of the patient. Within this framework psora is equated with the inanimate kingdom, sycosis with the plant, syphilis with the animal and the cancer miasm is classified as belonging to the human. One pillar of this approach is the assertion that 'we know there is not much cancer in most animals'. This statement is at odds with the extensive experience of the veterinary profession, certainly in the domesticated Western environment. Clinical practice shows that animals and humans react in similar ways to challenges and medication, which is what would be expected, both from their common biology and the model suggested in this book.

Limits of Imbalance within the Model

Inherent in the concept of balance is the consideration of what will happen when the limits of tolerance for that balance cannot be maintained and are then exceeded. Within the model of the miasms being presented here it is imperative that the integrity of the triangle is maintained at all times. If the activity of one miasmatic function is increased, represented by a lengthening of the appropriate side of the triangle, there must be corresponding adjustments in the lengths of the other two sides to compensate for this. (For the purposes of the model the changes in the angles are not important.) Similarly, a corresponding adjustment must be made if there are increases in the functional intensity of two of the miasms, with the greatest reduction in activity falling on the third. However, beyond a certain point, the integrity of the triangle cannot be maintained. Thus in the body the activity of any miasm to excess will result in a corresponding reduction of the other functions. In the early stages an increasingly precarious balance will be maintained, though with a decreasing degree of fluctuation and adaptability.

Finally, if the influence of any one miasm continues to increase, it will be impossible to maintain any semblance of the functional balance that is vital to life, and death will ensue. This is seen in cases of malignancy, where initially it is the increasingly active sycotic and syphilitic miasms that produce the pathology, although the normal processes of homeostasis can be maintained to some extent. As the condition worsens, either the sycotic or syphilitic force will come to predominate, depending on the exact nature of the growth. This leads either to the conversion of normal functional tissue into non-functional tissue, or to the destruction of vital tissue without replacement. In either case homeostasis cannot be maintained and death is inevitable.

Chapter 4

The Newer Miasms

The Relationship with the Basic Miasms

When miasms are discussed clinically there is soon talk of other miasms than the three that have been considered up to now. The Tubercular and Cancer miasms are widely recognised as clinical entities and others, such as Aids, are also postulated (Choudhury, 1992; Fraser, 2002). Sankaran, the influential Indian homeopath, has introduced the idea of up to ten miasms in total. There is no doubt that these influences exist, so how do they relate to the basic concept of the model presented in this book, and are they all of the same kind?

To understand this it is necessary to go back to the basic functioning of the body. The three fundamental types of physiological function that have been discussed, namely production, removal and control, correspond to the origins of the three Hahnemannian miasms of the original theory. However, as was indicated in Chapter 2, these three underlying activities form the basis of all body reactions, and hence are all that are necessary for the body to maintain itself in all circumstances of both homeostasis and response to challenge.

All the newer miasms are defined as clinical entities, not in terms of basic physiological function being linked to a range of symptoms, as is the case with psora, sycosis and syphilis, but rather by the symptom pictures that they produce. Thus it can be postulated that these symptom pictures arise as a result of the way that the body is functioning in various challenge situations *through the interplay of the three basic types of force.*

The Tubercular and Cancer miasms are the oldest of the newer miasms, and the clinical entities which they represent are well established as distinct and constant symptom pictures. This consistency implies that the three basic forces are acting together in a fixed pattern. In the same way that, for example, sycosis can always be recognised by excess of some sort, so the Tubercular and Cancer influences can always be recognised by the respective clinical pictures that they produce, including respectively the desire for change and the predominant theme of control (see Chapter 10 for further details). The range of symptoms that each of the two produces is different, which implies that the balance of the three primary forces is different in each, but the important point to appreciate is that the proportion of influence of each primary force is constant and the balance between them is fixed to a considerable degree. The tubercular balance is predominantly psoric and syphilitic, although the sycotic element cannot be ignored completely. In the case of cancer the major balance is sycotic and syphilitic, with psora being the least significant of the influences.

There is no absolute rigidity in the balance and some slight variation is possible between the individual forces, but the available range of movement is extremely limited compared to the potential of the perfect natural situation as discussed in Chapter 2. It is because of this slight residual flexibility that different remedies, with their own different individual balances, may nevertheless be described as having an association with one of the newer miasms, and, whilst being described in relation to that miasm, are also able to be identified in terms of the basic Hahnemannian miasms. Thus Phosphorus is described as a tubercular remedy because of the strong psoric and syphilitic elements in its make-up; Silica is similarly linked to some degree through its strong syphilitic component, whilst the high psoric influence in Calcarea Carbonica also corresponds to the tubercular pattern (Banerjea, 1993). Phosphorus and Silica are at the syphilitic end of the narrow tubercular range, whereas Calcarea is at the psoric end.

The term cancer as applied to the clinical disease is recognised as covering a range of pathologies of varying malignancy, yet the aetiological considerations involved in a homeopathic prescription of the nosode Carcinosin do not need to take account of the detailed pathology in a particular case. All that is considered is the broader classification of cancer. This variation of pathologies is another expression of the small but definite range of change in the balance that is seen in the miasm (see Chapter 5). Once this nearly complete stability has been established they may be classified as *mixed miasms* as opposed to being a *mixture of miasms*, which latter is the situation in chronic disease arising as discussed in Chapter 3. The tubercular and cancer miasms have reached this state of being mixed miasms.

A Recent Interpretation of Miasms

More recently, a different approach to miasms has been developed by Sankaran. In addition to the five already mentioned, namely psora, sycosis, syphilis, tubercular and cancer he adds firstly an acute miasm, and then introduces the concept of a further four, typhoid, ringworm, malaria and leprosy.

The relationship between the acute and chronic nature of individual diseases, and hence the relevance of the idea of an acute miasm, has been discussed in Chapter 3. Sankaran himself states: 'I have found that acute states can exist independent of the other miasms even for a long time', which can be interpreted as indicating a fundamentally different state to the other miasms. The other four are identified in terms of their relationship to the original Hahnemannian concepts. Thus typhoid is described as representing a state between the acute and psoric miasm, ringworm as being between psora and sycosis, malaria between acute and sycosis, and leprosy being linked to the tubercular/syphilitic end of the spectrum. (It is interesting to note that Hahnemann equated leprosy with the origins of psora rather than the more destructive manifestations associated with syphilis.)

Thus the two factors which are significant in defining these new concepts are firstly the symptom picture that is displayed, and secondly the make-up of that picture relative to the presenting picture of the basic miasms of psora, sycosis and syphilis. This implies that the physiological underpinning of the concept goes back to the three fundamental forces that cover all the body's reactions. Each of these newer concepts will have its own individual balance of those forces, but the important point is that the proportion of influence of each activity is different in every one. It is because of this difference that they can be recognised as distinct clinical entities, and defined by reference to the three basic forces. This linking of these newer concepts to the underlying basic functions represents a general view of the progressive dynamic of the disease process.

Within the understanding of the nature and function of miasms as presented in this book, the body's response to any disease situation must, by definition, involve all three of the basic physiological activities. It is the changing balance between these, as a disease process progresses, that is being expressed by the Sankaran classification. As he himself expresses it: 'We must remember that the miasms are only a classification; what must be cured is the disease state.' Allied to this is the idea of a progression of miasmatic dominance through life, with the acute miasm being seen as a major influence in the early years, the psoric influence during youth and adolescence, followed by sycosis in middle age, progressing into syphilis in old age. When considering the make-up of the individual remedies, Sankaran incorporates the acute miasm in an individual remedy's miasmatic pattern in addition to psora, sycosis and syphilis. Increasingly the term 'pace' is being used in relation to the Sankaran system, rather than miasm, as being a more appropriate way of reflecting the dynamic state of the disease process. This distinction is useful in appreciating the difference between the established newer miasms of tubercular and cancer and these more recent concepts.

The essence of any miasmatic state is a certain loss of flexibility in the responses that the body is capable of making to the challenges that come its way. Sherr reiterates this pre-eminence of function in both the health and disease situation when he says in his *Dynamic Materia Medica – Syphilis* (2002): 'In health people [and animals] are free to respond with any possible verb [function]. In pathology they are confined to a single function that indicates loss of freedom.' With psora, sycosis and syphilis – the *mixture of miasms* situation – although there is a predominance of one or more of the miasms and hence some loss of flexibility, there is nevertheless still considerable ability to adjust to circumstances and, with correct treatment, the possibility of restoring the original versatility. With the *mixed miasm,* as found in the tubercular and cancer states, the three basic forces have become more rigidly fixed, and hence a mixed miasm tends to act as one force with its own peculiar characteristics.

Because essentially the Sankaran model envisages a progression, either through life or disease, this implies a flexibility and adaptability to circumstances that is missing from the true miasmatic state. The states described as typhoid, ringworm, malaria and leprosy represent various less fixed transitional stages along a progression of disease. Clinically, they can be used as an aid to remedy selection by indicating the point along the progression that the patient has reached, but the basic miasms, which may be thought of as the major milestones along the way, offer wider implications and opportunities for treatment than the intermediate stages. If either an individual or a population gets stuck in one of these transitional stages for too long, then theoretically a new mixed miasm could be formed. It would, however, require exposure to the triggering challenge over a considerable period of time. The term *fixed miasm* is sometimes used to describe these transitional stages, but they are different to the combinations of the basic miasms under discussion here.

Other Claims to Miasmatic Status

The tendency to recognise new miasms with increasing frequency can lead to further unnecessary complication in a subject where there is already more than enough confusion. In this instance the problem goes back to the original misinterpretation of the miasmatic theory and the consequent implied connection with infective agents, which has created confusion over cause and effect.

The most recent development of this trend has been the identification by some of an Aids miasm. The view has been expressed that because Acquired Immuno-Deficiency Syndrome is a venereal disease, therefore Aids is a true new basic miasm (Choudhury, 1992; Fraser, 2002). This, of course, perpetuates the idea that the venereal diseases of gonorrhoea and syphilis are the direct root cause of the miasms sycosis and syphilis, which is too simplistic an interpretation, and does not accord with Hahnemann's perception. Two nosodes have been produced in connection with the infection, the major one using blood from an infected person. The other, known as Immunosin, has been developed in South America using the sperm of an HIV-positive patient. However, the fact that a nosode has been prepared does not automatically imply that a separate miasm exists. If that were the case, innumerable miasms would constantly be being added to with every new infection – which is clearly absurd, and is not happening.

The clinical picture of Aids has strong connections with the syphilitic miasm. This is supported by the aetiological link that has been well established between syphilis as the conventional disease and Aids as a clinical syndrome (Coulter, 1987). The appearance of tumours such as Kaposi's sarcoma and oral squamous carcinoma (Irwin, 1988; Finnegan, 1988) in the symptom picture are indicative of the miasm. Sankaran describes Aids as 'syphilis in disguise', and Sherr (2002) quotes modern treatment of syphilis with inappropriate antibiotics as being a major factor in the rise of Aids. The view has also been expressed (Strange, 1988) that it is primarily a tubercular manifestation, due to the incidence of tuberculosis that is seen in patients and the close match of many of the symptom pictures to Tuberculinum.

Any reaction to an infection, or vaccination, is sometimes being called a miasm. However, there is a vast difference between a reaction to vaccination or any other challenge and the creation of a miasm. This is not to say that such reactions are not serious and very undesirable, but it does not of itself represent a miasmatic state. Vaccinosis, although cited by Burnett (1884) as a miasm on the grounds that it creates a diseased state in an initially healthy body, is certainly a truly homeopathic chronic state, and therefore the miasms are involved, but the exact symptom picture that appears in an individual case will be as a result of the total interaction of both the miasmatic nature of the challenge and the miasmatic make-up of the subject (Saxton, 2005). Vaccination is generally regarded as a sycotic challenge to the system due to the creation of a reticulo-endotheliosis (Fortier-Bernovillie, 1934), and also as a suppression because of the abnormal and incomplete disease response that it produces (Saxton and Gregory, 2005). However, the clinical syndromes seen in practice following vaccination are not always mainly sycotic but are influenced by the inherited miasmatic pattern of the subject. Auto-immune disease, which is predominantly a syphilitic manifestation, can be produced by vaccination, and a causal link between Immune Mediated Haemolytic Anaemia and vaccination has been shown in dogs (Duval and Giger, 1996). See also Case 6, page 95.

It cannot be emphasised too strongly that in the author's opinion, although (homeopathically) all chronic disease is miasmatic, not every chronic disease is a new miasm. Equally, not every reaction following vaccination is a chronic reaction. Thus the aggression and/or the irritation around the base of the tail that is often seen following rabies vaccination in dogs and cats is not indicative of a rabies miasm, but of an acute reaction to the attenuated rabies virus. It has been said that '[it] is called the rabies miasm because it seems to be associated with the disease or with the vaccine for the disease' (Hamilton, 1990), but in the author's view this is more a definition of the causal link of the syndrome rather than of a true miasm. The cause of aggression in an animal is sometimes described as 'chronic Rabies', but this is chronic in the purely conventional, not the homeopathic, sense. In a truly miasmatic sense, aggression is most likely to be based in sycosis. Mention has already been made in Chapter 3 of Hahnemann's classification of Rabies as a 'half-acute' rather than a chronic miasm.

The type of definition quoted above in connection with the so-called rabies miasm has been applied to other infectious conditions. Influenzosis has been described as a miasm (Gutman, 1962), and in the animal world there is occasionally talk of a distemper miasm. Interestingly, there is not talk of a hepatitis nosode nor, in cats, a leukaemia nosode (in felines leukaemia is a viral infection). In the view of the author, distemper has been singled out because of the encephalitis and tertiary nervous signs sometimes associated with the disease. However, this is not sufficient to justify its classification as a miasm. The basic objections already discussed in relation to Rabies apply equally to these other cases, and it is worth reiterating that a causal link is not sufficient on its own to justify the title of a miasm. Equally, the variations that are seen between individual cases of vaccinosis in both humans and animals are greater than would be the case if vaccinosis were a true mixed miasm.

Treatment Implications of Mixed Miasms

The presence of a mixed miasm has implications for treatment over and above those that apply to conditions that only involve mixtures of miasms. The difference is that in cases involving mixtures of miasms, although the three basic forces are in a form of balance, albeit abnormal, each miasmatic influence still has an independence from the others and can be modified individually. Any such modification following treatment will of course result in the balance changing, and a different miasm may become predominant as an entity in its own right. In contrast, with a mixed miasm present, although a balance exists, the potential flexibility of that balance is lost; hence the effect is that a mixed miasm tends to act as one force rather than a combination of three forces. However, the essence of normal life and health is a fluctuating balance between the three complementary forces that represent the three basic physiological processes necessary for continued health and existence. Once the scope for fluctuation and adaptation is reduced, the ability to maintain a normal internal environment is compromised, and potentially the effect of this will be felt throughout the body.

In many ways the mixed miasms represent the greatest restriction on the free movement of the basic forces essential for health. In the Sankaran model, the tubercular and cancer miasms (the mixed miasms of this book's model) are placed towards the end of the progression; and the very fact that the ability for progression is envisaged in the earlier stages as being greater than towards the end implies an increasing loss of flexibility as the disease process evolves. Thus it is that many of the most serious and obstinate conditions met with in practice are often connected to the mixed miasms. The fixed nature of the patterns must be broken up if at all possible if real progress in a case is to be made. In reality, because of the fixed nature of the force in the mixed miasm, neutralisation by means of an opposite and similarly fixed force (the appropriate mixed miasmatic nosode) is often all that can be achieved. This has implications for the treatment of clinical conditions involving mixed miasms, such as cancer. This is discussed further in Chapter 6, and is where some of the greatest indications for the appropriate miasmatic nosodes will be found.

Chapter 5

Suppression

The Nature of Suppression

The concept presented in this book, namely that the miasms as clinical entities arise when the normal physiological functions of the body are blocked by inappropriate interference with the normal processes that they facilitate, leads on to the important question of what constitutes suppression in the context of both chronic disease and normal life.

Suppression is the theme that is central to the whole of the miasm story. As has been shown in Chapter 3, Hahnemann stressed throughout his writings the importance of its role in the creation of miasms as clinical entities. Paragraph 203 of the *Organon* states clearly the dangers of suppressing the external manifestations of disease. This was reiterated in his *Allopathy: a Word of Warning to all Sick Persons*, 1831 (*Lesser Writings*). Teixeira (2002) confirms the clinical observation of this phenomenon by homeopaths 'over the centuries', and also offers a possible explanation via known immune response mechanisms.

It is worth reiterating exactly what suppression involves. It may be defined as 'the sudden cessation or inhibition of a physiological phenomenon or the forcible removal of a disease manifestation before that disease is cured' (Mondal, 1998). Thus anything that interferes with the natural unfolding of the disease dynamic can result in the creation of a suppressive situation. Hahnemann wrote mainly about the adverse effects of suppressing skin eruptions, but this was only because of the clinical climate of his time. Not only was the aim to remove the skin rash at all costs in a case of 'the itch', but the treatment of the venereal diseases also concentrated in large part on the elimination of the exterior symptoms.

The greater range of interventions available to modern medicine unfortunately means that there is a greater potential for the suppression of the disease process at all levels, and it must not be thought that it is only the removal of skin symptoms that leads to suppression. Also, the continuous blocking of a normal and vital physiological process can lead to the same result. It is in this context that the development of agents for social convenience rather than medical need, such as the birth control pill, can lead to major problems, particularly in relation to the reproductive system, where the influence of the sycotic miasm can most easily become established (see Chapter 8). This may result, for example, in the establishment of an endometritis. The routine surgical neutering of animals also has implications here, and is further discussed later in this chapter.

Hering's Law, which is an expression of the dynamic of the curative process, states that the direction of cure is 'from within out', and from 'more important to less important organs'. Curative action is centrifugal, whereas suppression is centripetal. Anything that reverses or halts the centrifugal direction of the body's response is suppressive. The finding of 'from above downwards', although an integral part of the Law of Cure, is perhaps not of such great importance when considering the question of suppression – it is most relevant once the curative process has been thrown out to the skin. Nevertheless, the reappearance of old symptoms during the course of cure emphasises the importance of allowing the whole process to proceed uninterrupted if true healing is to be achieved. The working back of the whole 'dis-ease' process represents an important aspect of genuine cure in chronic illness. The inappropriate treatment of re-emerging symptoms can halt and reverse a beneficial reaction and lead to more suppression. It must always be remembered that this applies just as much to sensation as it does to pathology. The use of analgesics to control muscle pains or headaches that re-emerge during treatment can be just as suppressive as the use of agents to stop a reappearing diarrhoea.

Suppression is a major concern in the aetiology of chronic disease. However, it is possible to create a suppressive state, and hence a chronic disease, by the continued or repeated use of inappropriate treatment for acute disease. Even apparently purely external conditions, with an immediately obvious external cause, such as burns, have a systemic dimension. Palliation of conditions that are essentially curable will finally create a suppressive state.

The Mental Dimension

Since the three basic influences of production, removal and control that underlie the normal functioning of the body are active in both the physical and mental spheres, it follows that interference with the normal mental processes of an individual can be as suppressive as the inappropriate administration of drugs. The fact that the blocking of the natural mental processes of an individual may be in a sense a voluntary act (governed by the conventions of society or other influences) does not change the fact that the centrifugal direction of adjustment to challenge has been blocked. The link between the mental state and physical illness is now increasingly recognised in all medical models, but what is not universally appreciated is that the mental and physical processes are different sides of the same coin and function interdependently. Thus it is not, as the conventional model maintains, simply the case that external stress, acting as an external challenge, produces a state of mental depression which in turn acts on, and depresses, the function of the immune system. It is rather that the same response to the challenge of the stress is being seen throughout the whole patient simultaneously, and manifesting in different ways according to the level of the body in which it is allowed to occur. Hahnemann stressed that there is no such thing as a purely local condition, but that there are always systemic aspects to the situation. In Paragraph 186 of the *Organon* he states that 'Maladies of any import whatsoever, which have been inflicted on the body from without, draw the entire living organism into sympathy.' This applies just as much between the mental and physical planes as it does between different levels of the physical dimension. If the mental symptoms are properly addressed and allowed expression, then the patient's system is able to follow the natural direction of cure. If not, then the outward direction of flow is blocked. The 'dis-ease' remains and spreads within the other parts of the body, resulting in the manifestation of physical symptoms.

Emotions such as grief, anger, resentment and jealousy, if not allowed adequate and appropriate expression, will cause the body to react in this way, driving the process inwards. What is appropriate will, of course, vary with the individual, and may not require overt expressions of emotion: the important thing is that such expression as occurs is natural. It is from the suppression of normal emotional outlets that the mental aetiologies of disease arise, expressed in the repertory as the rubric 'Ailments from …'.

The treatment of mental illness by the use of medication can also lead to suppression. Hahnemann observed that apparent improvement in the mental state of patients frequently led to the development of physical symptoms which were absent whilst the mental symptoms were present. Paragraphs 210 to 230 of the *Organon* discuss the interrelationship between mental and physical disease.

The Progress of Suppression

Hering's Law states that the more superficial the organ, the less important it is for the individual's survival, and the aim of the direction of cure is to remove disease away from the vital centres. Suppression counters that aim. It does not however mean that all suppression inevitably leads to death, although some suppression can lead directly to life-threatening conditions, such as the development of malignancies. In many cases the result is the creation of a state which does not carry major risk to life (although some may be present), but which nevertheless represents a state of considerable disease. The seesaw balance between asthma and eczema has been well recognised for centuries and represents such a situation, with the asthma improving as the eczema worsens, and vice versa.

By the same reasoning, the tendency of the curative process to move a disease outwards is still naturally present in many cases where there is a miasmatic imbalance. This is why sycotic and syphilitic symptoms may be found on the skin (see Chapter 6). But in cases where there is suppression, the different miasmatic influences are seen to follow different routes inwards. To understand this it is necessary to look briefly at the origins of the body's development. It must also be remembered that the more deep pathology there is in a case, the greater the influence of sycosis and syphilis will be found to be. This is because psora, being linked to the control function of the body, manifests more as a purely functional upset (see Chapter 7).

During the development of the body, the tissues and organs arise from three primary germ layers, the ectoderm, mesoderm and endoderm (also known as the entoderm). The ectoderm, the outermost of the three layers, is the origin of the skin (and associated structures such as glands and nails), the mucous membranes of the mouth and anus, the entire nervous system and the external sense organs. The middle germ layer, the mesoderm, forms the basis of the muscles, connective tissue, bone and cartilage, blood and systems, kidneys and gonads. The endoderm, the third and inner layer, accounts for the epithelium of the respiratory tract, the digestive tract and the bladder.

The most superficial and, from the point of view of survival, least vital organ is the skin. Hence in many cases the appearance or reappearance of symptoms involving the skin represents the correct direction of the curative process. When a skin reaction is suppressed, the disease process will be directed inwards. If the major miasmatic influence in the disease is psoric, the organs that will be next attacked are those others that arise from the ectoderm, and the result is an upset to the nervous system and its function. If there are sycotic or syphilitic influences in the skin reaction, suppression will lead directly to the involvement of organs derived from the mesoderm and endoderm. In general terms, sycosis will involve the endoderm, and syphilis the mesoderm (Henneman, 1996). The nature of the overriding physiological functions of these organs is such that they reflect the tendencies and characteristics of these two miasms. But these deeper structures are the ones that are most important for the body's survival. Thus it is, that although finally any miasm may be present in any organ, as disease is increasingly driven inwards, so the more destructive and pathological miasms attain a greater prominence, with a corresponding worsening of the disease state. Conversely, as a cure proceeds there may be the appearance of the less life-threatening effects of the other miasms in less vital organs.

Miasms in Neoplasia

Neoplasia is essentially the multiplication of abnormal cells, and a prominent feature is that the growth is uncontrolled. This represents the sycotic miasm, where the regulated production of new tissues has been tipped over into an excessive production. Thus, by definition, it would follow that a strong sycotic element is involved in all tumour formation. In tumours that are classified as benign, the cells, although dividing abnormally, still retain a high degree of differentiation, and in these cases the sycotic miasm is very prominent. At the other end of the scale are the highly malignant growths, a marked feature of which is the undifferentiated nature of the cells. This breakdown of order in the cells may be regarded as the influence of the syphilitic miasm; and as the clinical definition of tumours moves from benign to malignant there is a corresponding change in the balance of the miasmatic influences. A wart represents the simplest of sycotic growths. The psoric element is present in the loss of control that allows the development in the first instance, with the absolute minimum of syphilitic activity. (It must, however, be remembered that continuing wart production associated with other sycotic symptoms in a case, such as metritis or cystitis, may represent an attempted exteriorisation of the deeper disease.) Similarly, lipomas and fibromas are predominantly sycotic. Carcinomas and sarcomas on the other hand show a high level of both sycotic and syphilitic activity. The rapid proliferation of the cells is sycotic, whilst the uncontrolled spread (loss of boundaries) and the destruction is syphilitic. The more malignant a growth is, the greater is the predominance of the syphilitic miasm. In between there is a gradation of pathologies depending on the exact miasmatic balance that is present. In general terms, the more undifferentiated cells there are present in the tissues the more destructive, i.e. the more syphilitic, is the growth.

It is therefore both possible and desirable to consider histopathological reports from the miasmatic point of view, and thereby to obtain an additional dimension in the interpretation of a case.

Suppression plays its part in the aetiology of neoplasia just as much as in any other condition. Since it is the production and removal functions which become especially activated in the body's response to challenge, it follows that suppression of those natural activities will tend to produce conditions representing miasms associated with those functions.

Preventive Suppression

In modern conventional medicine interventions are increasingly undertaken either to prevent what is perceived as a risk of more serious disease, or to control and change normal physiological functions for non-medically justified, or purely social, reasons. In the first group are found procedures such as the surgical removal of warts and apparently benign lumps 'in case they turn nasty'. The error here is that there is no understanding of the directions of both disease and cure as understood in the homeopathic world, and no awareness that inappropriate treatment of an exterior phase of a disease can result in it being driven inwards. The presence of warts, lipomas and cysts may be regarded as no more than a cosmetic inconvenience, and dealt with accordingly, rather than being recognised as part of a broader disease process. Even if the worst consequence of the removal of warts is the appearance of more warts, this is often regarded as nothing more than a further cosmetic inconvenience. In the animal world the removal of anal glands in carnivores falls into the same category – as modified sebaceous glands they are part of the skin's excretory function, and so-called 'anal gland trouble', with repeated impaction and/or infection, is in fact only part of a wider picture.

There will, of course, be occasions on which such interventions are valid for a variety of reasons. But such indications should not blind the practitioner to the wider health implications of the situation, thereby allowing suitable supplementary treatment to be provided as appropriate in order to balance the case.

In the second group the major area of concern is the modern approach to, and methods of managing, the physiology of reproduction. In all species these procedures are undertaken for social or commercial reasons, rather than involving the application of strictly medical criteria. They take the form of either increasing, or more usually and worryingly, decreasing or stopping completely, the activity of the reproductive system. Whether the procedures are surgical or chemical, each may lead to untoward effects, although the chemical manipulations are potentially the more hazardous since the reproductive organs remain intact and therefore a possible seat of consequent pathology. In contrast, their surgical removal means that any effects will be seen elsewhere in the body. Although the mammary glands – the one remaining reproductive organ – may be affected, the overall effect is usually to produce symptoms in a more diffuse form. There is also a difference in the way the procedures are applied between species, with permanent suppression being more common in animals, whilst temporary or intermittent control is practiced more in humans. Although the less interference with function there is, the less the potential for harm arises, nevertheless all such procedures should be viewed with caution.

Although these methods are more often aimed at the female, in the veterinary field the male is also involved to some degree. But whatever the species or sex, the procedures represent a form of suppression, with all the potential consequences that this entails.

It must be remembered that the normal rhythms of reproductive physiology, as well as being geared to a particular biological function, are also part of the overall balances of the body. If the system is absent, and therefore non-functional, a new functional balance must be created. If the system is still present but is not being allowed to function normally, then the establishment of that necessary new balance becomes more difficult, especially if the suppressed system is in a young subject who is either still maturing or at the height of reproductive activity. Also, the normal cycles of function through the various reproductive or post-reproductive phases are part of the body's *natural* processes and progressions, the blocking of which is potentially harmful to overall health. The regular discharges of the female reproductive system may have a role in the maintenance of the normal balances in the body, acting as a 'safety valve' where the full functions of pregnancy and birth are not followed through. False pregnancy in canines in some ways fulfils the same function.

It is widely known in veterinary work that the use of chemical contraception, either by injection or orally, to suppress the first oestrus can lead to a lack of subsequent reproductive activity, or, if it is still present, to reduced fertility. This, in miasmatic terms, is a manifestation of a psoric effect, the result of blocking the activity of the ovary before it becomes fully functional. Once full activity of the reproductive system has been established, the effects of suppression become potentially more serious, and the continued use of contraceptive procedures often results in the manifestation of more sycotic and syphilitic symptoms. Chronic cystic endometritis (pyometra) is essentially a sycotic condition and is being seen increasingly in young animals, where previously it was a condition of the more elderly un-neutered female. (Occasionally this is being seen after just a single use of a chemical contraceptive agent in animals where there is a latent sycotic miasm.) Chronic cystitis is another manifestation of the suppressed sycosis trying to find an outlet. Malignant mammary tumours are also known to occur as a consequence of the use of chemical contraception.

Continuous blocking of the function of an entire system may cause it to turn in on itself and create pathology. This is especially so when the biological function of that system is particularly strong. Mention has been made of the reproductive system being a major site of the physiological function of new tissue creation. When this is blocked it reacts by attempting to recreate the normal function (a form of secondary counteraction). This predisposes to the creation of the sycotic miasm, which manifests as the excessive production of new tissues and discharges as described above. Hering's Law describes the progress and direction of the curative process, but in the author's view the above examples show that there is another law, a law of disease, which states that 'the suppression of the normal function of a vital system will often drive that function inwards to become pathological *within that same system.*'

The menopause in humans is a function that is not shared with the animal species, but it must be remembered that this too is part of the normal reproductive physiology and that the completion of the process is part of nature's way of maintaining the necessary balance in the system. Interference with its working-through by the use of hormone replacement therapy can be just as much a suppression as the use of chemical contraception earlier in life, with similar potential consequences. A survey of over 46,000 women for between ten and sixteen years showed that those taking an HRT preparation had an increased risk of breast cancer, which was related to the length of time the preparation had been taken (Schairer et al, 2000). There were also variations in risk depending on the exact hormone preparation used, with mixed hormone preparations carrying the greatest risk. The paper quotes other studies with broadly similar results. Chlebowski et al (2003) and the Million Women Study (2003) have both shown increased risks of breast cancer of up to 26% in women taking HRT, plus increased risks of stroke and heart disease. Whilst the exact interpretations of these surveys have been questioned, it is clear that there are major biological effects linked to these medical interventions. To add insult to injury, an American study showed that there was no benefit in terms of lifestyle between women using HRT and those on placebo (Hays et al, 2003).

The other procedure carried out routinely in animals is the surgical neutering of healthy young females. There is a valid case for this policy, as both the medical and social consequences of not neutering can be extremely undesirable. Indeed, the policy of keeping entire cycling females without any attempt to breed from them could be regarded as a form of suppression in itself. But it must be borne in mind that the removal of the reproductive organs also removes a potential outlet for the sycotic miasm, which will if necessary find expression elsewhere. This is also a consideration following hysterectomy in the human. Indeed, the use of the contraceptive pill in patients already attempting to cope with chronic disease may constitute an obstacle to cure by blocking a natural body outlet.

As mentioned above, the mammary glands are an integral part of the reproductive system, and these may become involved as the only remaining outlet. The appearance of pathology in the reproductive system during treatment of another presenting condition may well be part of the curative reaction, and treatment of this new symptom without recognising it as part of the wider process constitutes a form of suppression. The routine castration of male animals does not have the same social imperative and is a practice to be deplored from the miasmatic point of view. Vasectomy, of course, does not interfere, from nature's point of view, with the functional integrity of the reproductive system.

Because of the widespread nature of the above practices, in addition to the generally suppressive nature of much allopathic and antipathic medicine, it is easy to see why there has been a vast increase in sycotic manifestations (e.g. cancer) in the present era and why it has now become a major miasmatic influence in chronic disease. The first response of the body to most challenges involves an increase of some function, for example inflammation and/or pyrexia. The suppression of these functions by medication will predispose towards the establishment of a sycotic miasm. It appears in many cases almost as though the eruption of the sycotic miasm allows the creation of pathology in tissues, providing the portal for its more destructive syphilitic cousin to enter and flourish, once the initial breakdown of normal physiology has taken place.

CASE 1: *Suppression and a blocked outlet*

An eight-year-old entire Old English Sheepdog presented on referral with an osteosarcoma in the lower third of the left ulna. She had been vaccinated as a puppy but not again until she was four years old, since when she had received annual boosters. She lived with her lady owner and another six-year-old Old English Sheepdog, with whom she got on well. She had suffered from arthritis for the previous three years and had been taking non-steroidal anti-inflammatory drugs, which were controlling the symptoms. Her oestrus (period) had been normal, at six-monthly intervals, up to twenty months previously, since when it had been present on only two occasions. There had been no other major health problems until the present troubles.

Two months prior to the homeopathic examination a small tumour had been removed 'as a precaution' from the penultimate mammary gland on the left side. No histology was carried out, it being declared benign on clinical grounds. Its appearance had not been linked to an oestrus cycle, the latest of which had occurred some four months previously.

Increasing lameness on the left front leg had initially been considered part of the arthritis, and the dose of non-steroidal anti-inflammatory had been increased accordingly. When this failed to relieve the situation a radiograph had been taken some two weeks prior to the consultation, which had revealed the osteosarcoma.

On a scale of one to ten, with ten representing complete non-use of the leg, there was a 6/10th lameness. Normally a friendly, outgoing, reasonably energetic dog with a good appetite, she had withdrawn into herself over the previous weeks, becoming less interactive with both her owner and the other dog, and had lost her appetite virtually completely.

There was a noticeable swelling on the affected leg immediately above the knee (the wrist in human terminology), which was hard, but not painful, to the touch. The lymph nodes were not enlarged. The radiograph showed extensive bony destruction of the lower ulna with minimal new growth on the surface of the cortex. The lungs were normal on auscultation and there was no cough.

The owner was induced to stop the anti-inflammatory drugs, and initial homeopathic treatment was with Aurum Metallicum on the basis of the depression, the diminished appetite, the presumption of increasing pain as indicated by the increasing lameness and the highly destructive appearance of the bone on X-ray. A 30c potency night and morning for five days was administered. This produced a clear mental improvement and the dog's appetite returned to normal, but there was no change in the lameness. Rather than repeating the Aurum, perhaps at a higher potency, it was felt that the underlying miasmatic aspect of the case, as indicated by the extreme destruction seen on X-ray, needed addressing more directly. Hence three doses of Syphilinum 200c were given in twenty-four hours, on the basis of the ongoing pain and the indication for Syphilinum in cases of osteosarcoma. (The reference in the materia medica is to osteosarcoma of the tibia: however, in animal work, due to the locomotor as opposed to prehensile function of the forelimbs, it is often possible to be guided by the function and utilise the descriptions and rubrics found under lower limbs.) This prescription was followed by Symphytum 30c night and morning for ten days, both as a local remedy directed at the pain, and also for its indication in sarcomatous tumours. This resulted in the complete restoration of her normal mental state and the lameness reduced to 3/10ths.

Towards the end of the course of Symphytum, a cystic endometritis developed, and without consultation the referring veterinary surgeon performed a panhysterectomy. Recovery was uneventful. The opportunity was taken to X-ray the leg again, which showed an increase in the new tissue around the lesion but no decrease in the destructive area. The homeopathic prescription was changed to Calcarea Fluorica 30c night and morning for five days, on the basis of its connection with bone integrity, its still predominantly syphilitic nature, the continued bony swelling around the affected area, and its complementary connection to Syphilinum. The mental alertness was maintained but there was a gradual worsening of the lameness over the next month until there was a 5/10th lameness. The affected leg was X-rayed again, and this showed that there had been further degeneration in the bone involved in the lesion. The prescription was changed to Hecla Lava, whose remedy picture shows it to be a syphilitic/sycotic remedy with lower limb pain in that picture, plus an indication in cases of osteosarcoma: a 30c potency was administered once daily for ten days. The worsening of the lameness ceased but there was no improvement.

Three weeks later the mammary tumour returned at the site of the previous operation.

This time, however, it was clearly of a much more aggressive nature than before and was quickly spreading into all the glands on both sides. Carcinosin 200c night and morning for five days stopped the spread. The limp had worsened somewhat and Hecla Lava 30c was reintroduced night and morning for one week. Further doses of Carcinosin 200c, night and morning for two days weekly, produced some reduction in the tumour size. Throughout all of this the dog continued to be mentally alert and playing with the other dog. Unfortunately one particularly exuberant play session caused her to be pushed off a two-foot high wall and land on the affected leg, resulting in sudden onset acute pain, but mercifully no fracture. However, the referring veterinary surgeon prescribed short-term steroids and re-introduced the long-term non-steroidal anti-inflammatory drugs in order to control what was regarded by him as a terminal situation. This introduced a suppressive element into the treatment regime, but with courses of Hecla Lava, Symphytum, Carcinosin and Syphilinum as appropriate, the situation was kept tolerable for some eight months, with additional steroids themselves being periodically prescribed by the referring veterinary surgeon. Finally a sudden worsening of the lameness and a complete collapse of the dog caused the owner to request euthanasia when she was *in extremis.*

Discussion

Due to the differences in approach and organisation between the veterinary and medical professions, the management of this case would not, of course, have followed the same pattern in the human sphere, but it demonstrates the dangers of the conventional mindset, and emphasises Hahnemann's view, expressed in Paragraph 74 of the *Organon,* that 'The life force is, in part, mercilessly weakened by these treatments and, in part (if indeed it does not succumb) it is gradually abnormally mistuned.' It is very much a tale of initial suppression, followed by aggravation of the condition due to blocking of the outlets through which the body was attempting to deal with the situation. The first precautionary surgery, undertaken with the object of preventing later troubles, in fact had the opposite effect, driving the disease inwards with a corresponding worsening of the miasmatic picture. The initial mammary tumour exhibited predominantly sycotic/psoric features with its apparently non-malignant nature, but the more inward manifestation, when it occurred, was clearly predominantly syphilitic with a lesser sycotic element. The initial homeopathic treatment resulted in a reversal of this, with the sycotic miasm becoming again the greatest influence and finding an outlet in the reproductive system. Suppression of this by the surgery caused a reversal of the healing reaction and the re-emergence of a syphilitic domination of the case. The reappearance of a mammary growth was not the return of an old symptom in accordance with Hering's Law. Rather, because of the blocking of the sycotic outlet as a result of the hysterectomy, the mammary glands were the only part of the reproductive system left to react. Unfortunately, due to the complete dominance of the syphilitic miasm by this time, the reaction was of an altogether different type to the initial involvement.

However, it is interesting to note that the recurrence started at the site of the previous surgery. Although no biopsies were taken, clinical experience suggested that histopathology of the second mammary neoplasia would have indicated an adenocarcinoma. Thus Carcinosin was indicated as the nosode of choice (Chapter 9), with Syphilinum being added later as the ultimate syphilitic remedy in an attempt to counteract the overwhelming miasmatic influence. The Hecla Lava and Symphytum were prescribed as local remedies for the osteosarcoma, both being remedies with a sycotic/syphilitic bias. The dog remained bright and lively throughout the latter stages and so it was not thought appropriate to repeat the Aurum Metallicum, as depression would be a major part of the Aurum picture in this type of case. An acceptable degree of control for a while was all that could ultimately be achieved.

Although it will never be known, it is reasonable to suppose that with suitable homeopathic treatment of the endometritis, which would have allowed the continued expression of the sycotic miasm and the further direction of the curative action outwards, and without the additional suppressive effects of the later orthodox treatments, a different outcome could have been achieved. The additional suppressive effect of the later steroids and anti-inflammatories was a further detrimental factor, and it is likely that the sudden collapse at the end was another manifestation of the disease process being driven inward.

CASE 2: *An active miasm*

A large four-year-old neutered male Dachshund presented with a chronic skin irritation affecting the head, chest, abdomen and the whole of the back of both hind legs. He had been acquired at six months of age from a breeder, purely as a pet, because he had an undescended right testicle that had failed to respond to conventional treatment. As a result he had been neutered at ten months old. He had been vaccinated and wormed routinely with no immediate apparent ill effects. The skin problems had started shortly after he came to the present owners. Its first appearance was under his chin but it quickly spread.

Initial conventional treatment was with medicated shampoos but these gave no benefit, and after several months systemic steroid therapy was instigated via tablets. This controlled the situation as long as the tablets were being administered.

When he had been on treatment for about a year he suddenly lost the use of his hind legs. The condition was painless and radiology revealed no spinal lesions. Complete continence was maintained. The condition was treated with non-steroidal anti-inflammatory drugs, and it slowly resolved. The steroid treatment was stopped coincidently at this time, as the skin condition was thought to be allergic in origin and treatment with antihistamines and shampoos was substituted for the steroids. The bathing gave temporary relief, but the owners did not feel that the antihistamines were helping to any great extent. This situation continued for around two years, with no recurrence of the back problem, and the skin being controlled solely by bathing.

On examination there was little to see on the skin except a thin, poor quality coat on the affected areas, and some scars, which appeared to be the result of self-mutilation. He would scratch until he bled, and the wounds were always slow to heal. There was no heat in the skin, but the ear canals would occasionally flare quickly and become hot, red and painful. Steroid-based ear drops were being used as necessary. There was no obvious problem involving the back at the time and the pedal reflexes were normal.

The dog was described as 'placid, gentle and laid back', indifferent to all except his owners, and liking heat and comfort. He was active but never moved very quickly, and was never keen to walk far from home. There were no obvious fears, he ate well but slowly, and drank normally.

Calcarea Carbonica 200c was selected as the initial homeopathic treatment, based on the temperament and physical appearance of the dog. Three doses in twenty-four hours resulted in a general increase in mental alertness and a considerable reduction of the scratching. A further similar dose was administered after three weeks when the improvement had stopped (although he had remained bright and alert in himself). This apparently resolved the condition. Five weeks later a sore developed on the dorsal aspect of the neck and the irritation returned to the legs. The sore was very irritant and moist with a sticky discharge. Graphites 30c night and morning for four days cleared it. After a month he was re-presented with his legs and abdomen red, hot and irritant. Sulphur 30c fitted the presenting symptom picture, and a dose night and morning for four days settled all affected areas. A similar flare-up six weeks later also responded to the same regime. Subsequently Sulphur in courses of ascending potencies up to 1M over the following nine months resolved the problem completely.

Discussion

This is a case that could be seen in any species. The pattern of psora runs through it, starting with the retarded development represented by the undescended testicle, although in all other respects development had been apparently normal. Reproductive development faults can also be syphilitic, and undescended testicles are usually psoric / syphilitic. However, there had been no other members of his litter with any problems, and a strong syphilitic influence would have been likely to have produced more widespread affects in the litter. As the skin problems had started before the neutering it was not a case of suppression by that procedure. The idiopathic paraplegia following steroid therapy is typical of a suppressed psora, and the resolution of that probably owed more to the stopping of the steroid therapy than to the non-steroidal anti-inflammatory drugs. Those may, in fact, have slowed the recovery. The dog appeared an obvious Calc. Carb. type, but in spite of the apparent good match and response, the situation was not completely resolved before other manifestations led to the use of other antipsoric remedies. Sulphur and Graphites are both antipsoric, with major skin symptoms in their pictures. Calc. Carb., while having a prominent psoric element, is also sycotic to a considerable degree. Thus the Calc. Carb., whilst appearing to be the simillimum, clearly did not address every aspect of the case. The subsequent eruption of symptom pictures matching other psoric remedies indicated that the psoric miasm was still active until treatment with those remedies resolved it.

The length of time required for complete resolution of the problems is consistent with Hahnemann's contention of the deep-seated and obstinate nature of miasmatic disease.

Chapter 6

Miasms as Therapeutic Tools

Perceptions of Miasms

Miasmatic prescribing can appear to be a separate activity, divorced from the search for the simillimum. In fact, considerations of the miasmatic influences in a case are part and parcel of the search for that perfect match which represents the totality of the symptoms. In South America a tradition of prescribing based primarily on miasmatic considerations has developed (page 11). In other parts of the world the miasmatic theory was for a while regarded as an historical anachronism of no practical use, and miasms have often been ignored in favour of methods based solely on repertorisation from the presenting picture.

However, repertorisation has its limitations, such as the tendency in many cases to overemphasise the polychrests and the under-representation of some remedies. Cases occur where the process of repertorisation does not produce the desired remedy and an alternative strategy is needed. Both repertorisation and miasmatic prescribing have their own validity, but a willingness to combine the two as appropriate is likely to yield the best results. Hahnemann writes in Paragraph 2 of the *Organon* of the need for the 'lifting and annihilation of the disease in its entire extent'; and in *Chronic Diseases* he stresses that 'he [the physician], therefore, must first find out as far as possible the whole extent of all the accidents and symptoms belonging to the unknown primitive malady.'

The importance that miasmatic factors are given will always vary from case to case, but their influence is an integral component of all disease processes, both acute and chronic, and they represent a very important aspect of the totality of the symptoms. J.H. Allen, in his *Chronic Miasms*, considered that the strange, rare and peculiar symptoms which Hahnemann stressed as so important were, in fact, essentially miasmatic, and produce their spectacular results because they reach down to the deepest levels of the individual. In chronic disease, consideration of the miasmatic patterns will often enable the prescriber to see the essence of the case. Even in acute conditions there are miasmatic considerations that can assist in the selection of the correct remedy, including situations when a genus epidemicus is sought. Their main usefulness, however, lies in the field of chronic disease.

Paragraph 5 of the *Organon* exhorts the physician to 'find out the data of the most probable occasion of an acute disease, and the most significant factors in the entire history of a protracted wasting sickness [chronic disease], enabling him to find out its fundamental cause. The fundamental cause of a protracted wasting sickness [chronic disease] mostly rests upon a chronic miasm.' Paragraph 7 emphasises that 'it must be the symptoms alone by which the disease demands and can point to the appropriate medicine for its relief, along with regard for any contingent miasm', and later 'the totality of symptoms must be the most important, indeed the only thing in every case of disease, that the medical-art practitioner has to discern.' Hahnemann was led to the miasms, not by a complete failure of his prescriptions to act, but by the limited action that his apparently well-selected remedies were having in a proportion of cases, and also by the fact that an apparent cure was sometimes followed by the emergence of a new symptom picture representing, in conventional terms, a new disease. A correctly selected remedy will inevitably bear a relationship to the miasmatic situation at the time of its selection, but that situation may change as the case progresses and new aspects of the dynamic disturbance are exposed. The underlying miasmatic balance will determine the true nature of the overall 'dis-ease'. Thus the consideration of the miasmatic factors involved often provides a means of getting to the heart of a case.

Miasms may also constitute a block to the normal working of the body's disease response, and one of the advantages of the theory is that it offers a way of identifying that block and either overcoming or controlling it. The impression is sometimes given that if there is a strong miasm present then the best that can be achieved is palliation. While it is true that the presence of an unresolved miasm in a case may prevent a cure, it is by no means correct that it must remain unresolved in all situations. It is possible to overcome these detrimental influences, but successful prescribing in such cases requires the consideration and incorporation of the miasmatic features of the case together with all other aspects. Indeed, it is in these situations that a high priority must be given to the miasmatic features in the symptom picture. Although at various stages of a case the prescribing strategy may be changed as seems appropriate, regard must always be had to the overall picture.

Recognising Miasms

In most cases the presenting signs and symptoms, if explored fully, will contain elements of all three miasms. However, in many cases there will be a predominance of those arising from a particular miasm. Hence it is important to be able to recognise the various miasmatic influences, and an overview of a case will often reveal a pattern of symptoms that points clearly in the direction of a particular miasm. There may be, for example, a marked time modality in all symptoms, a generalised over-production of all tissues, the marked involvement of certain particular organ systems, changes in the quality of nails, claws or hooves, or the nature of discharges. Sensations in humans may provide information that is unavailable with animals, such as feelings of tightness of clothing or modalities attached to eating. The patterns so revealed can point to the major influence in the case at that time. Consideration of the pathological nature of the condition being treated is also of value, and an appreciation of an overriding theme of deficiency, excess or destruction in the disease is a useful pointer. In this context the use of laboratory and radiological data can be helpful. Investigation of the family history may reveal a definite pattern that has been inherited by the patient. In a one-sided case the initial use of this approach may aid in the subsequent choice of a remedy by broadening the perspective of the presenting picture. That does not mean that the relevant miasmatic nosode should be used automatically, but it can be indicated where there is a clear connection with a particular body system, or other strong indication of a particular influence. In other situations, a remedy that both reflects aspects of the symptom picture and also has a strong connection to the appropriate miasm is likely to be the most effective.

The Miasmatic Overview

The symptom picture of a case when it is first presented will reflect the miasmatic balance at that time. This will be the result of the miasmatic inheritance of the patient, together with the experiences and challenges to which they have been exposed. A correct prescription will take account of this, although the strength of the miasmatic picture can vary widely. The picture may be so clear as to immediately suggest a remedy with a strong miasmatic link, such as Mercury to syphilis or Thuja to sycosis. Alternatively, further clarification may be sought by repertorisation, and this will result in narrowing the choice to a smaller number of remedies. The final selection here will as usual involve more detailed consideration of the remedies, and it is at this point that an appreciation of the miasmatic pattern of the case can be of help. Thus if the choice were to be between Calc. Carb., Sepia and Baryta Carb., a definite indication of sycosis in the case would, other things being equal, tip the selection in favour of Sepia, as this is the most strongly sycotic of the three remedies under consideration. The remedy pictures as set out in the larger materia medicas will often contain information about the miasmatic orientation of the remedies.

In the author's opinion, the rubrics of 'psora', 'sycosis' and 'syphilis' found in the repertory are not themselves particularly useful for repertorisation. They are really too large, having around two hundred remedies in each, and the majority of entries are in the first degree. The rubric for psora has only two remedies, Sulphur and Psorinum, in the third degree (Schroyens, 2004). Although there are rubrics for tuberculosis and cancerous affections, these are not the same as rubrics for the respective miasms. Using other features of the case as sources for smaller, more balanced rubrics will yield a more accurate result. The 'miasmatic rubrics' are generally only of use when being referred to as part of the subsequent elimination process rather than as main rubrics, and are useful as a source to establish the miasmatic connections of remedies. However, consideration of the miasmatic pattern of a case can be of help in the selection of suitable rubrics for repertorisation. If an overview of the case shows a particular miasmatic pattern, then rubrics which reflect that pattern are often the most appropriate.

Once a successful first prescription has been given, the patient will present with an altered symptom picture, and in assessing the significance of this, consideration of the miasms can be of help. This is not the place to consider all the possible permutations of the patient's response, but some are more indicative of miasmatic activity than others.

The emergence of new symptoms that cannot be attributed to the remedy

This may indicate a change in the miasmatic balance of the case, and is further discussed below.

A temporary improvement in all of the main symptoms with a subsequent regression

The way forward here, having reassessed the appropriateness of the prescription, will usually be to repeat the remedy but in a different potency, usually higher. If this either fails to act or again produces only a temporary response of similar duration, then the possibility of a miasm acting as a block to curative action should be considered. If the duration of the response to the second prescription is considerably greater than with the first, then a further alteration of the potency should be tried before a change of remedy.

The use of a miasmatic nosode such as Psorinum, Medorrhinum, Syphilinum, Tuberculinum or Carcinosin in these circumstances is a way to unlock the case and then allow other remedies to complete their action. One of the bowel nosode group of remedies may also be of use, as these have strong general connections to chronic disease and the miasms (see Chapter 10). The author's experience is that the potency selected should initially be moderate, with a later increase if necessary. Alternatively, the LM potencies may be used.

Some symptoms have abated but other pre-existing symptoms have become more prominent

The remaining prominent symptoms will now often point towards a particular miasm, and this should be given great weight in the selection of the next remedy. The appropriate nosode may be given if it fits the remedy picture, but the selection of a remedy that has a strong relationship with the now clearly presenting miasm may be the best way forward.

If a number of remedies have been employed but none has had a significant or lasting effect, the use of a miasmatic nosode should be considered. The use of too many remedies in a chronic case can be detrimental, and miasmatic prescribing will help to avoid this, by concentrating the remedy selection on the primary deep-seated imbalances in the case.

The initial prescription in a case is usually of a remedy other than a miasmatic nosode. Unless there is a clear symptom picture pointing to a particular nosode, miasmatic prescribing is usually something for the second and subsequent prescriptions, after the effect from previously prescribed remedies has been observed. The main exceptions to this are when, in spite of the careful selection of several remedies, a successful first prescription cannot be made and nothing seems to have any effect; or where there is no clear remedy picture but a definite miasmatic pattern. Here a miasmatic nosode as above may be employed to start the case. As already stated, in these circumstances a moderate potency should be employed initially.

The other exception is when there is advanced pathology linked to a mixed miasm, as in the case of cancer. More will be said about this later, but the use of a miasmatic nosode in conjunction with other remedies will often give the degree of control that is necessary in these cases.

The Miasmatic Progress of Cure

As already discussed in Chapter 5, as disease is suppressed and moves inwards, the effects of the sycotic and syphilitic miasms become more apparent, with the appearance of increasing amounts of frank pathology such as growths and ulceration. Hering's Law operates in the opposite direction to this, with the curative process trying to move the disease process outwards, away from the deeper and vital organs. However, the effect of Hering's Law is not always to get rid of the miasmatic effects completely right at the start, but to move them into less important regions and if possible to find an outlet for them. In this process the presenting pathology may well be relieved while new pathology linked to the same miasm appears in other organs. Thus on occasion, following a successful prescription, new symptoms can arise that are apparently unconnected with the original condition (see Case 1, page 59).

As was discussed in Chapter 3, any remedy will itself have influences in its make-up that represent antimiasmatic properties. If it is correctly chosen in a case based on the presenting symptoms, then the balance of those properties will bear a relationship to those symptoms, but it is likely to represent only the similar rather than the simillimum. Such a strong antimiasmatic prescription can result in a change in the miasmatic balance and thereby affect the type of symptoms that subsequently appear. However, it may well not get to the heart of the case; as a result it does not necessarily mean that the influence of the previous dominant miasm has been eliminated, but only that the balance has been changed. It may be necessary to return later to that aspect of the case and approach it at the deeper miasmatic level of the miasmatic nosode. Looking at the developing symptoms in a case from the miasmatic point of view can aid substantially in helping sense to be made of what is happening in the patient.

In chronic disease there will often be one particular miasm that is most prominent. A possible starting point in such a case is to first treat the presenting miasmatic picture with a remedy selected on the simillimum principle that has the appropriate antimiasmatic action. In Paragraph 209 of the *Organon* the instruction is given that 'based on these symptoms [i.e. those being exhibited by the patient], the physician starts the treatment by selecting the (antipsoric, etc.) medication that has the utmost possible similarity of signs to those of the disease.' If there is a clear pattern of the activity of a particular miasm across a range of systems, then the corresponding miasmatic nosode may be considered as a starting point. If there is no clear miasmatic pattern presenting initially, a remedy selected on the presenting picture may, as discussed above, result in the emergence of a clearer picture. Alternatively, a prescription based on only the psoric symptoms in the case may be employed. By thus addressing those aspects of the case representing a deficiency of function, such as dryness of the skin, constipation or a general aggravation from cold, the whole can be given a stimulus which can result in a clearer picture emerging. In cases with little or no clear presenting picture, Hahnemann suggested the use of Opium, which is a strong antipsoric remedy, to stimulate the system.

The result of a successful prescription will be a changed symptom picture, and the next prescription should be based on that picture. This change will often be due to a changed balance in the miasms, and so a further correct remedy will reflect that new balance. In some cases the miasm will still remain the same, although the symptoms will represent a different aspect of it. This prescribing strategy is repeated through all the changing manifestations of fluctuating miasmatic balances until the symptoms of the 'dis-ease' are exhibited predominantly in the skin.

Hahnemann, in both *Chronic Diseases* and the *Organon,* states that the final stage in the curative process is the reappearance of psoric symptoms. It is well known that sycotic and syphilitic symptoms, such as greasiness, pigmentation or ulceration can be found on the skin, and the reappearance of them in the course of treatment may represent the functioning of Hering's Law. This would imply a functioning immune response rather than a deficient reaction. On the other hand, the fact that sycosis and syphilis are still active does mean that there is still some imbalance and lack of adequate control. In practice this means that not all skin symptoms appearing later in a case should automatically be treated with antipsoric remedies (see Chapter 7). It is only when all symptoms of sycosis and syphilis have left the skin that the end can be considered to be in sight.

Hering's Law and miasmatic influences involve both the physical and mental levels, and have relevance for the treatment of mental illness (and behavioural problems) as much as for the purely physical. These former are often examples of 'one-sided' diseases, that is those cases exhibiting only a small number of prominent symptoms within one system of the body. Hahnemann, whilst regarding them as having mainly an underlying psoric cause, stressed the importance of taking into account the full miasmatic picture, and treating them in the initial acute stage with remedies other than the major antipsorics (the so-called apsoric remedies). In Paragraph 222 of the *Organon* he states that 'a patient who recovers from an acute mental and emotional disease by means of apsoric medicines should never be regarded as cured. On the contrary, once the acute outbreak has passed, the patient should be given, as soon as possible, a continued antipsoric (and possibly antisyphilitic) treatment in order to entirely free him from the chronic miasm.' The exact choice of remedy will of course be made by consideration of the presenting symptoms, but the miasmatic pattern is an important aspect of that picture.

The Mixed Miasms

Conditions involving mixed miasms (Chapter 5) can be among the most difficult to treat, and it is here that the miasmatic nosodes are the most use. Indeed, they could be said to be essential in these conditions. Because of the unified but still unbalanced nature of the functional response, as discussed in Chapter 3, these are the cases where it is most difficult to deal with the basic miasms one at a time. The symptom picture does not change in response to treatment to nearly the same extent, due to the fixed interrelationship of the forces. The approach mentioned above of initially concentrating on the psoric symptoms may be successful here, due to the general stimulus to the system that this can provide. However, where there is advanced pathology as a result of a mixed miasm it is often the case that control via regular use of the appropriate miasmatic nosode is the best that can be achieved. This has proved successful in the treatment of a range of cancers in humans (Ramakrishnan and Coulter, 2001), and the author's experience is that the same approach is valid in animals. This control will also involve the concurrent use of other remedies selected on the basis of the presenting picture. As the use of the nosodes is potentially long-term, care must be taken with the choice of potency. Some authorities (Ramakrishnan) favour a basis of 200c with regular plussing to minimise the chances of an aggravation, although other potencies will be required in individual cases. This is an area where the LM potencies have great potential.

Miasmatic Considerations in Disease Prevention

As mentioned in Chapter 3, the concept of the inheritance of a load of miasmatic 'baggage' has been utilised to devise eugenic treatments in order to clear such a load before birth. Similarly, miasmatic nosodes have been recommended as a means of preventing the development of disease states in those individuals whose family history indicates an increased likelihood of clinical problems occurring (Ramakrishnan). Thus it may be thought advisable, where there is a strong family history of clinical cancer, to administer Carcinosin as the appropriate miasmatic nosode at intervals of a few months purely as a preventive. If patients with such a family history are receiving treatment for other apparently unrelated chronic conditions, they may still benefit from the occasional dose of Carcinosin as an intercurrent remedy. Likewise, Tuberculinum has been recommended as a means of pre-empting the onset of seasonal respiratory disease.

The objection can be raised that this is not true homeopathy, as the individuals in question are not ill and are therefore not exhibiting any symptoms – there is no suffering for the prescription to be similar to. However, what is being advocated here is not the routine administration of the nosodes to every individual, as is the aim in the case of a vaccine being used for a population-based preventive programme. In every case, whatever the presenting condition, where a deep homeopathic prescription is being arrived at, the family history should be considered as part of the totality of the symptoms. (The fact that often in veterinary work a detailed family history is not available does not lessen the desirability of having one.) A strong history of major miasmatic imbalance in a case increases the likelihood of any challenge converting the latent force into an active one. In effect, the potential patient is in such a state of miasmatic disease as to be suffering from a permanent pre-disease state.

Cases of malignant neoplasia which have been 'cured' by conventional means involving the removal or destruction of the lesions will, of course, still retain the miasmatic make-up that was present before the disease manifestation. This is another indication for the use of miasmatic nosodes in a preventive role, as such cases may still be considered to be at high risk because, from the miasmatic point of view, a major underlying factor in the disease process has not been addressed. Nor can the miasmatic considerations be ignored where the neoplasm is diagnosed as benign (see Case 1, page 59).

The 'Miasmatic' Nature of Challenge

Within the framework of this discussion, it may be postulated, as discussed in Chapter 3, that all remedies have an antimiasmatic make-up that consists of a balance of the three functional forces. These three biological forces, which are the basis for the miasms, have their equivalents in the rest of nature. That balance, which is fixed, varies from remedy to remedy, and some are more strongly inclined towards particular miasms than others. The antimiasmatic nature of a remedy is a reflection of the original energetic nature of the source substance, activated into a medicinal form by the process of potentisation.

Further, from this it follows that all substances from all kingdoms have an energetic potential that mirrors the influences that are recognised as clinical patterns in homeopathy. Although Chinese Traditional Medicine is a separate discipline from homeopathy, that too has the concept of the basic elements of life being intrinsic in nature as well as being present in the body. This further implies that all challenges, whether they are from an infectious agent or any other source, have an energy balance that can resonate with the miasmatic and pre-miasmatic forces in the body. The better the resonance, the greater the susceptibility of the patient to the remedy will be – and it is through this resonance that mixed miasms like the Tubercular miasm are established.

This resonance will pertain in relation to any challenge, and if the force of the challenge is strong enough, either by single or repeated exposure, it will impose its nature on the body. This imposition will not necessarily be a total reflection of the underlying miasmatic balance in the body, but may be a temporary effect reflecting more the 'miasmatic' nature of the challenge. The underlying balance will be reflected to some extent in the overall chronic disease picture, but the temporary resonance with the forces of the challenge may dominate the immediate acute symptom picture. The balance will revert to its previous state once the challenge has been correctly dealt with and is over, but if the treatment is not correct, or the challenge persists, then longer-term problems will be created. Thus repeated exposure to either a massive, or repeated smaller, doses of radiation, which is intrinsically a destructive force, will provoke a destructive response from the body in the form of a malignancy.

This consideration of the energetic potential of a challenge can be of use in understanding the miasmatic balance of a remedy. For instance,

Lachesis is derived from snake venom, which is both cytotoxic and neurotoxic, its purpose being to destroy and paralyse. These functions equate to the syphilitic and psoric miasms, and in the remedy these two are indeed the major influences.

Non-physical events can also act as challenges and set up reactions in the body, and an appreciation of the energetic nature of those challenges can on occasion help in remedy selection. Thus mild or moderate damage to the body of a tendon requires essentially a routine maintenance task. Help via a tissue-related remedy such as Ruta Graveolens, with its psoric (weakness) and sycotic (new growth) emphasis is probably all that is required. But the tearing of a tendon insertion is a more violent happening, requiring a more vigorous (and 'violent') response. Such an injury will be more likely to respond to a more syphilitic remedy such as Phytolacca.

Miasms as therapeutic tools offer advantages in that they can give help in both remedy selection and in providing a perspective to a case, enabling treatment to progress from one logical point to the next. This applies whether consideration is given to the underlying patterns of the traditional miasms, or to the more modern dynamic concepts of the 'paces' of the disease process. Through miasms it is possible to follow and understand the body's reactions to its disease, and by recognising the dynamics of the situation, to intervene more effectively.

CASE 3: *Physiological suppression*

A six-year-old entire female German Shepherd Dog presented with three mammary tumours each about half the size of a golf ball, two in the hindmost glands on the right hand side and one in the penultimate gland on the left. They had appeared over the previous two months, firstly on the right, and all were hard and painless on palpation. The dog was otherwise fit in herself, there were no enlarged lymph nodes, no cough, and her lungs were clear on auscultation. The possibility of surgery was discussed and rejected.

She was the only dog in the household and was described as friendly and liking company, but disliking too much physical petting and holding. She was generally nervous, with an especial dislike of noise and hatred of thunder and fireworks. Her appetite was normal, her only craving being for apples. Thirst was described as above average with large amounts being taken at one time, and a preference for drinking when the water was straight from the tap, and therefore cold. She sought heat but was happy to be out in the cold if playing or walking.

She had received initial and booster vaccinations up until the age of three but none since then, and there had been no health problems up until around four years of age.

Oestrus intervals had been variable between six and nine months, but the season (period) had been normal when it occurred. At three-years old she had been mated and produced three healthy puppies with no difficulties. At the beginning of the next oestrus she had been given proligestone (Delvosteron) as a chemical contraceptive to suppress it and this had been routinely repeated six months later. No further contraceptive injections had been given and she had not exhibited oestrus since then.

She had subsequently developed bilateral otitis externa, with the right ear being the worst affected. This had been treated with a topical mixed steroid and antibiotic preparation. This gave relief, and there had been occasional flare-ups since then, which had all been treated in the same way.

Treatment was begun with a homeopathic preparation of Delvosteron, prescribed on a 'never well since' basis. The 30c potency was selected because of the nature of the pathology present, and a dose night and morning for five days was given. Three weeks later all the tumours had reduced in size by about a quarter and there was a definite soft tissue swelling around them. There was no sign of oestrus, but six days after finishing the tablets there had been some urinary urging with traces of blood for thirty-six hours. No further treatment was given at this stage, and two weeks later the soft swelling had cleared while the tumours were unchanged. Scirrhinum was then prescribed, three doses being given in twenty-four hours. The general nervousness, dislike of noise, large thirst for cold water, love of heat and desire to play pointed towards both Phosphorus and Scirrhinum, and the fact that the first growths appeared on the right, and continued to be worst on that side, was a factor against prescribing Phosphorus.

The decision was taken to use a miasmatic nosode derived from mammary malignancy as part of the treatment, and the hardness of the growths indicated Scirrhinum rather than Carcinosin. This was followed by Phytolacca 30c night and morning for a week, chosen because of the hardness of the glands and the predominance of the right side in the picture, with a lesser spread having occurred to the left. This resulted in a softening of the tumours but no change in size. Phytolacca 30c was repeated once daily for ten days. A month later all the tumours had reduced to half their original size, and the associated tissue swelling had returned. There had been signs of oestrus but only for around seven days rather than the full three weeks of a normal canine season, and the vulval region had remained swollen. Delvosteron 30c was repeated, this time three doses in twenty-four hours, as it was felt that the original obstacle to cure arising from the contraception was still a factor in the case. This resulted in the vulva returning to normal.

Following this hoped-for removal of the obstacle, Scirrhinum 200c was repeated in the same twenty-four hour dosage pattern as previously. This produced a considerable painful oedematous swelling around the mammary area. Apis Mellifica 30c, three times daily for two days removed this. The tumours had now shrunk to a third of their original size and had become even harder. Conium 30c was administered night and morning for five days on this indication, giving a further reduction in tumour size. At this stage the otitis returned to the right ear, with thick, black discharge. There were also signs of further vulval irritation, although no discharge could be seen. Elaps 30c resolved these symptoms. Conium 30c once daily for seven days produced only a slight further change. No further treatment was given, as the owner was not prepared to face the prospect of further reactions. The residual tumours have remained as they were at the end of the treatment. Periodically there were some signs of oestrus but with no set time pattern, and a full season never develops. The residual tumours have remained as they were at the end of the treatment, and she continues otherwise normal and happy in herself.

Discussion

As with Case 1 (page 59), this situation would probably have been approached very differently in the medical as opposed to the veterinary context. The possibility of surgery was rejected on two counts, firstly on the homeopathic principle of not removing an external expression of disease unless absolutely necessary on welfare grounds, and secondly due to the owner being unwilling to subject an apparently otherwise fit dog to surgery if it could be avoided.

This case shows suppression of two fronts: firstly a physiological suppression of the oestrus and secondly a therapeutic suppression of the resulting otitis. Scirrhinum was chosen rather than Carcinosin because of the symptom picture, especially the hardness of the growths. The painful reaction that occurred following the last administration of the remedy was also consistent with the remedy picture. Ideally, further attempts should be made to completely normalise the oestrus, and hopefully this restoration of the normal physiology would allow complete resolution of the residual tumours, but the chosen policy of 'let sleeping dogs lie' precluded that.

Within the model, the physiological suppression resulted in the initial psoric effect of a lack of ovarian function, thus allowing the creation of an altered miasmatic imbalance. Because of the involvement of the reproductive system in the suppression it was the sycotic miasm that subsequently manifested, as an ear problem, following the natural direction of cure. Further suppression of that resulted in a deeper manifestation of sycosis, which appeared in the mammary glands due to the natural tendency of the miasm to involve the reproductive system. The initial and subsequent treatments using a homeopathic remedy based on the conventional prescription (tautology) were attempts to restore the previous balance. The fact that this was only partially successful indicated the possibility of a mixed miasm, with a significant syphilitic component. Hence recourse was made to the miasmatic nosodes. Both Phytolacca and Conium have significant syphilitic and sycotic features in their pictures, namely a destructive tendency and the production of hard growths, fitting in with the pattern of the lesions in this case.

CASE 4: *A changing picture*

A four-year-old neutered female cat was presented with colitis and a history of skin problems. She had been in the same home all her life and had been neutered as a routine at six months of age. She was essentially an indoor cat by her own choice and used a litter tray, although she had access to the garden via a cat-flap. She was vaccinated regularly against everything possible and there had been no acute reactions to the procedure. The first sign of trouble had been the appearance of irritant scabs on her back at around two years of age. This had been diagnosed as 'fleabite allergy', which was treated with systemic steroids, and a regime of continuous flea control was instigated consisting of both systemic and local components. This had been followed conscientiously ever since, and although no fleas had ever been seen, the skin had continued to give occasional trouble that was settled by injections of steroids as necessary.

The owners had seen occasional bouts of diarrhoea throughout the cat's life, which never seemed to upset her. However, about eighteen months prior to the consultation she had suffered her first attack of severe abdominal pain, accompanied by diarrhoea. The diarrhoea contained much mucus and blood throughout it all, and its passage provoked severe straining and the passing of offensive flatulence. Interest in both food and drink had been lost for some thirty-six hours and she had become completely apathetic, with no interest in her surroundings, wanting only to remain in her bed and sleep. Her abdomen had been tense and she had resented pressure on it. These attacks had become more frequent and were now happening approximately every six or seven weeks. They had been treated with various antibiotics and steroids. At the time of the consultation she was on a low maintenance dose of steroid, but with little beneficial effect. She was recovering from an attack at the time, and the stool was still loose with mucus and blood, and some straining during passage.

The cat was described as being of an independent nature, with little interest in either other animals or people. She would accept holding and petting for a short time from people she knew well, especially the female owner, but she would then insist on running off, although there was never any aggression linked to her desire to escape. She disliked noise and would disappear if the owners shouted at each other. There was no clear heat preference indoors, but if she did go outside she would not lie in the sun. Appetite and thirst were described as normal, but she would not of choice eat dry food. She loved cheese and milk, which she was given on occasion. In spite of the involvement of the bowels in the condition, ingestion of these did not precipitate an attack.

The steroid was stopped, the dose being low enough for this to be done quickly without any risk. Mercurius Solubilis appeared indicated because of the blood and mucus in the stool during an attack and the intense straining that accompanied its passage, and a 30c potency was administered night and morning for four days. The attack settled quickly and was followed by a further mild attack five weeks later. Merc. Solubilis 30c was again administered, resulting in a quick resolution. Thereafter there was no more colitis but the motion was periodically a bit loose, although the cat was not upset by it and remained mentally alert and, according to the owners, 'her usual self'. The scabs on the back returned and were extremely irritant. The coat was greasy to the touch with some hair loss, which appeared to be a genuine loss rather than being mechanical due to the scratching induced by the pruritis.

Natrum Muriaticum 200c, three doses in twenty-four hours, was prescribed. The mental and general symptoms fitted the picture of the remedy, as did the local sign of the greasy skin. The scabs regressed but the irritation remained. The Nat. Mur. 200c was repeated after one month, resulting in the remaining scabs resolving completely. The coat lost its greasy feel and became dry with some dandruff, and both its quality and quantity improved. It was now felt that the only hair loss was self-inflicted, as the intense irritation remained, and there were two or three sores present which would be made to bleed by scratching. The now poorly-defined symptom picture, together with the fact of self-inflicted bleeding sores, led to the selection of Morgan Bach as the indicated remedy, with its major action on the skin and intense irritation. A 30c potency was administered night and morning for three days. This completely stopped the irritation within one week. There was a return of the irritation two months later, without any scabs, and Morgan Bach 30c was again administered. There was no sign of any further bowel problems. The irritation disappeared quickly once more and there has been no trouble since then.

Discussion

This case could apply to any species. It demonstrates how the deepening of the disease process following suppressive treatment, in this instance by steroids to control a skin condition, can be reversed by appropriate homeopathic interventions. Although painful abdominal conditions tend to be sycotic, due to the excessive muscle contraction that produces the spasm, there was clearly more in this case than just a straight sycosis. The initial presenting symptoms revealed a syphilitic component in addition, as shown by the quantity and distribution of the blood in the motion, which was present all the time and appeared to be a result of primary, active bleeding, rather than being induced as a secondary effect by the spasm and straining.

Although no investigations were carried out, the indications were towards an ulcerative colitis as a result of the syphilitic influence, rather than the lesser, more passive bleeding that would have been seen due to involvement of the other two miasms. The straining and the mucus indicated sycosis. Treatment with Mercury, a predominantly syphilitic remedy with some sycotic (mucus production) element, selected on the basis of the presenting picture, produced a return of the sycotic involvement of the skin (the scabs and the grease represented an increased production). Further treatment selected on a wider constitutional picture changed the skin to a more psoric state with less pathology and the more pure functional upset of the dry skin with irritation. The sycotic and psoric miasms are both well represented in

Nat. Muriaticum and Morgan Bach. Natrum Muriaticum is, however, the more sycotic of the two, and hence the order in which they were required, with the psoric element coming to the fore later in the case. This is an example of well-chosen remedies reflecting the miasmatic balance of the patient at the time of their prescription, and their use resulting in changes to that balance as the whole case moves towards a cure.

Chapter 7

Psora

Basic Concepts

Psora is in many ways the most difficult of the miasms to understand. Hahnemann in *Chronic Diseases* called it the 'mother of all disease', and a 'hydra-headed monster'. Although ideas about its nature have changed over the years, that original concept remains valid today. This is because of its central role in the regulation of both homeostasis and the response to disease. In *Chronic Diseases* Hahnemann made two claims for it; firstly that neither of the other miasms could obtain a hold without the presence of psora, and secondly that it was the miasm which was capable of causing the maximum of functional upset with the minimum of pathology. In *The Substance of Homoeopathy* Sankaran shows how a sycotic state can emerge from an underlying psoric one.

The normal control of the body's physiology has two components. There is the day-to-day maintenance of the internal environment. Then there is the regulation and adjustment of the productive and removal functions as appropriate in response to challenge situations. In addition to the regulation of immune function in the conventional sense, this also implies the orchestration of the direction of cure as outlined in Hering's Law, and it will be seen how vital this is in the working-out of any disease process.

Within the suggested model it has been postulated that in any disease situation there will be elements of all three primary functions present in the body's response. Given that the physiological requirements of homeostasis require a central and controlling role over the other functions, as discussed in Chapter 2, it follows that when either or both of those functions manifest as miasmatic influences, this must be as a result of a loosening of the control over the physiological functions that precede them. The initial loosening of the control may well be intentional and desirable in response to a challenge, but once it is over there is then a failure to re-establish the necessary order. The essence of psora as a miasm is now thought of as deficiency or failure of function (Ortega, 1980). Loss of control may be viewed as a form of deficiency, and within this framework Hahnemann's first claim in *Chronic Diseases* – that the presence of psora is a prerequisite for the establishment of the other miasms – can be seen to be upheld.

The other way in which a deficiency can also be produced is through excessive control, and this excessive control, when it is present, is a function of the psoric miasm. This results in an undue influence on organs with a corresponding reduction in their function, and a resulting upset in the homeostasis of the body. But this does not initially involve the development of pathology. If the malfunction continues for long enough then pathology may appear, due to the activities of either or both of the other two influences. Hahnemann's first concept of the necessity for psora to be present is represented by this over-control, but his second concept in relation to psora, that of a purely functional upset, is intrinsic to its nature.

Psora can be viewed as corresponding to Grauvogl's Carbo-Nitrogenoid constitution, which is characterised by a deficiency of oxidation of the blood, resulting in his interpretation of an imbalance of nitrogen and carbon in the system. The tissues do not absorb enough oxygen, resulting in poor metabolic function and hepatic weakness. It is commonly thought of as 'the itch disease', its name being based on the Hebrew word for itch. In Hahnemann's time the most common manifestation of this was known as scabies, although it must be remembered that without the assistance of modern diagnostic tools this term probably included a whole range of dermatological conditions. In fact, Hahnemann did not so much associate psora with the presence of scabies as with the latter's suppression by the use of topical preparations on any skin lesion. His concept envisaged more than just a superficial irritation.

The Terminology of Psora

The Hebrew word *tsorat*, linguistically linked to the origins of the word *psora*, was known to Hahnemann and in fact conveys his concept much more accurately. It had been used in Hebrew to describe both the plague and leprosy, the implication being of uncleanness. Leprosy was identified by Hahnemann as a previous manifestation of psora, and from which he appears to trace its development, through various stages, into the scabies of his time. The meaning of *tsorat* is a fault, stigma, groove or pollution, and from the beginning this was an essential part of his concept of psora. In *Chronic Diseases,* his first mention of psora is not in relation to the skin, but is concerned with the reoccurrence of disease. He states that such reoccurrence 'would be especially the case whenever a seemingly cured disease had for its foundation a psora which had been more fully developed.' He then goes on to link the development of disease to the presence of a skin eruption in the case history, especially if suppressed, but then returns to a definition of the underlying 'malady which may be called by the general name of psora: i.e. against the internal itch disease with or without its attendant eruption on the skin.' It appears to the author that the concept of psora has connections to the increasing modern understanding of the nature of many deficiency and genetic diseases.

Later Interpretations of Psora

In the meantime there have been other ideas concerning the nature of psora. One interpretation of 'fault' led to the connection of psora with the religious philosophies of moral inadequacy and original sin as expounded by Kent and others (Chapter 1). It was held that the presence of this inherent spiritual weakness allowed the establishment of other influences that resulted in the physical manifestation of disease. A variation on this theme is that the current concentration of many modern societies on external gratification rather than seeking internal individual peace is the cause of the basic imbalance in the system, and that the basic animal desires are being given too much free expression (Miles, 1992).

On a purely physical level H. A. Roberts (1868–1950), basing his interpretation on Boenninghausen's, with his list of antipsoric remedies, considered that psora could be equated with problems involving the assimilation and balance of elements in the body, notably what are now regarded as trace elements. Similarly Edward Bach (1886–1936), through his work with the bowel flora and bowel nosodes, initially considered the lack of function and stagnation associated with psora to be due to enterotoxaemia, and regarded this at one time as being synonymous with psora, and hence with the root of all chronic disease. However, although failure of both absorption and utilisation of nutrients is psoric in nature (Banerjea, 1993), Bach's initial interpretation confuses cause and effect, and his subsequent work with the Flower Remedies was the result of his change of view as to the true nature of disease. The action of the Flower Remedies is directed towards correcting the negative emotional and mental aspects of a case, many of which are psoric in nature, such as the doubts and indecision of Cerato, Honeysuckle's attachment to the past, Wild Oat's indication in passive individuals who have not responded to other treatments, and Gentain's depression following grief and bereavement. (Hahnemann considered that the major trigger for the flaring of latent psora was grief.)

In *The Substance of Homoeopathy* Sankaran equates psora with the basic struggle of life, both internally and in relation to the outside world. Internally there is a constant battle to maintain the balance of the functions that is forever threatening to be lost. Externally it is equated with change and loss, and there is the perception of a constant struggle to maintain the equilibrium and restore the status quo. This interpretation envisages an 'acute' miasm that is active before psora appears. As discussed in Chapter 3, the acute miasm can be considered as akin to the situation described by the diagrams in Chapter 2, and psora becomes the struggle to recreate the perfect balance. However, as has been shown, it is a struggle that is often doomed to failure; and, as the battle begins to be lost, so the other miasmatic influences come increasingly to the fore. While it is true that there is an element of change and adaptation in psora, the development of this view of miasms leads to the idea of a progression through life from psora via sycosis to syphilis. Although such a pattern has some general validity, it does not appear always to be the case, and the implied linear deterioration is not necessarily so. Throughout life all three forces will continue to act in some degree, and the balance will vary with the individual.

Clinical Manifestations

The essence of psora may therefore be regarded as either a deficiency of function or a failure of the regulation of function.

Clinically this will appear as those conditions that are described as 'hypo', and those that are associated with nutritional deficiencies and imbalances. These nutritional abnormalities are not those caused by malnutrition due solely to inadequate dietary intake, but rather those that arise as a result of functional upset. With psora there is an inability of the body to respond to situations, and this manifests as feebleness or inadequacy, deficiency, reduction, paralysis, atrophy and inability. Mentally this shows as restlessness, anxiety and oversensitivity, with feelings of being alone and unsupported. There is much mental activity but very little to show for it. There is an inability to marshal ideas and think a situation through. The slightest stimulation results in many ideas being produced, but they cannot be controlled and ordered into positive action. This can appear in the form of many ideas being produced and talked about at great length for a short time, and then dropped as another interest is pursued. Lack of control of the thought processes results in mood swings and anxieties about the individual's ability to cope with a situation, and these may develop into phobias and delusions.

Concerns about being able to cope may extend to feeling inadequate to meet the challenges of the day, and hence many of the fears are at their worst in the morning. Minor occurrences and upsets can produce disproportionate feelings of inadequacy. Fears of illness and death are marked, as being situations in which the individual feels particularly helpless; and any illness is perceived as being potentially fatal. Dreams are vivid and reflect the fears and anxieties of the type, and nightmares are common. Sleep is often disturbed and unrefreshing. There is a tendency to substitute activity for achievement, which shows as both a physical and mental restlessness. Activity is undertaken at an excessive level for a short time. This then ceases because the concentration cannot be sustained and, at the same time, the psoric individual is easily exhausted by the effort.

At the other extreme there can also be weakness of memory and low mental activity. The lack of confidence, linked with much superficial mental drive, leads to dissatisfaction combined with an unwillingness to do anything about changing a situation. The situation may arise when an individual knows what needs to be done but is still unwilling to do it. There is an overriding lethargy. The whole mental approach results in a person who is consumed by their own concerns and reactions. These are not the natural 'leaders of men' nor, in animal terms, the pack or herd leaders. Vertigo in a range of situations is a common symptom, often triggered by emotional factors. Headaches tend to be unilateral and are accompanied by nausea and upsets to the functions of the senses. Mental conditions will improve when physical illness appears. Conversely the anxieties of psora are increased by the suppression of skin eruptions, which is consistent with Hahnemann's view that mental illness is basically psoric.

Although the time modality is not as marked as in the other miasms there is a definite tendency to < before noon and > afternoon. Physiological discharges will produce amelioration, as will the appearance of skin eruptions. Pathological discharges often have a foul smell to them. Heat regulation tends to be poor, and so there is both a desire for heat and an amelioration from it, with a corresponding aggravation from cold. The weakness of the control of heat regulation can also result in much and easy perspiration, and this can occur on the slightest exertion or even at rest. Conversely, there may be a lack of perspiration. Flushes of heat with redness of the skin are seen, and in those animal species that do not possess sweat glands, and hence do not perspire naturally (carnivores), there may be spells of unaccountable panting (this is different to the situation in humans and other species which do normally perspire). The need for stimulation can lead to a desire for both sweet and sour things and seasoned food, although bland food is often preferred. Indigestible things may be sought, and there is a general aversion to milk. Fats are often desired even though they cause digestive upsets. Hot food and drink is the ideal. The usual dietary desires and aversions may be reversed during fevers.

The skin is dry and looks unclean and unkempt, often with a strong smell. In animals the coat is dull and lifeless. Irritation without any primary lesions is a feature. This may be intense, and scratching gives only temporary relief whilst resulting in self-inflicted wounds. Skin eruptions are rough and non-infected, with dandruff. The hair tends to be thin and fall out easily, and early greying may be seen.

Heart problems are functional rather than pathological in nature and have a definite link with mental symptoms. They are both caused by, and produce, much anxiety and fear of death; emotional upsets are a major aetiology. Feelings of fullness, constriction and congestion are experienced within the cardiovascular system, along with sharp pains. The pulse is usually full, although bradycardia is seen and there may be an irrational feeling that the heart is about to stop.

The upper respiratory system is a major seat of psoric activity. Burning pains and feelings of constriction are typical, and conditions tend to occur in the winter. There is generally little mucus production and the cough is dry. Respiration is slow and usually shallow, and cyanosis is a feature.

The alimentary system is characterised by good to ravenous appetite, in an attempt to overcome the deficiencies of the system, although loss of appetite will also be seen. Poor peristalsis leads to poor digestion. There may be a taste of burning in the mouth. Hunger is often seen in the morning, especially around 11 a.m., and at times there will be an urgent and overwhelming desire to eat immediately. Conditions are generally improved by eating. In spite of this, the underactive digestion produces feelings of fullness and bloating and being easily satiated. There is bloating and flatulence throughout the system, and overeating produces many symptoms associated with the abdomen. Constipation is common, and apart from the feelings induced by eating, bowel conditions are generally painless. Some patients may feel better when constipated, although constipation is often associated with pains in other areas of the body. Diarrhoea, when it occurs, is worse in the mornings.

The urinary system shows patterns linked to deficiencies such as incontinence and inability to pass urine, even though the bladder is full. Weakness of bladder control leads to involuntary urination linked to coughing or similar convulsive movement (barking in dogs produces the same situation).

The psoric influence renders females particularly susceptible to external influences during menses and pregnancy (and also often to remedies). The inexplicable dietary cravings that are seen during pregnancy are psoric in origin. During pregnancy there are inevitably major changes in the hormone balances in the body, and increased nutritional demands. These may put a severe strain on homeostasis, with the results described above. Sexually there is irregularity of oestrus and menses in females, impotence in males, and a general low libido in both sexes. Puberty may be delayed and fertility is generally deficient.

The lack of lesions associated with manifestations on the skin is mirrored in the other systems where the emphasis is on loss or distortion of function with no or minimal pathology. The lack of proper control and balance within the system results in inappropriate responses to stimuli. One aspect of this is a tendency to produce a fever at the slightest challenge. There is a general sensitivity to external stimuli and a particular sensitivity to the new moon. Slow development generally, sluggish metabolism, and muscular weakness also reflect the miasm. The head is often small in a psoric individual.

There is usually a sensitivity to strong tastes and smells, although as the state progresses the external senses tend to become deficient. Abnormal noises will be heard in the ears, and this is often linked to a marked sensitivity to noise.

Suppression of psora drives it primarily into the nervous system. As with all else connected with the miasm, the effect here is one of functional upset rather than the establishment of pathology. This is one aspect of the 'empathy' of the control influence for all body systems concerned with homeostasis, and this extends to other systems as well. Prolonged suppression leads to effects beyond the nervous system, particularly in the endocrine system.

Hering's Law and Psora

It must not be assumed in chronic disease that just because there is a reaction on the skin, it is the psoric miasm which needs to be dealt with. Part of the physiological function of the body is to throw a disease process outwards in accordance with Hering's Law. A sycotic or syphilitic manifestation is thus exteriorised as the result of a normal reaction. Skin conditions that show lesions such as hypertrophy, excessive secretions, ulceration and so on are not indications of the psoric miasm. On the contrary, they are indications of the activities of the other miasms. Their appearance on the skin represents a normal response to the disease process and is part of an active immune response. In many psoric cases the only lesions seen will be either self-inflicted, the result of normal physiological functions that have gone out of control (e.g. inflammation), or other external factors or agents. There is a marked lack of suppuration in pure psoric skin cases, and when it is seen the discharge is thin and watery with a strong odour. The skin surface will be either dry or with a serous discharge. The vesicles, when they occur, provide an outlet for the disease, and it is when these are suppressed that the internal manifestations of psora are seen. Failures of normal function, such as hair loss, will also be seen.

The influence of psora will also be seen in cases that initially fail to produce an adequate exteriorising response to challenge. In these there will often be no external manifestation, or at best a small, continuous problem such as an intractable otitis externa. Overcoming the psoric influence in these cases can result in more extensive skin lesions appearing, but these are the result of the sycotic and/or syphilitic influences present in the case, and are not due to the psoric miasm.

The role of suppression in the creation of miasms cannot be emphasised too strongly.

Right from the beginning of his investigations Hahnemann realised that the appearance of much internal disease was associated with the suppression, at some time in the past, of skin lesions, and this was clearly stated in the early pages of *Chronic Diseases*. Even in those cases where the 'cause' was an external infection, the treatment of these conditions by external applications led to a suppression of the body's natural route of healing. In those cases where the condition was misdiagnosed, and there was in fact an existing internal condition concurrent with the external manifestation, such suppression would lead to an even more serious internal disease.

Psora and Allergy

At first sight it may seem odd to claim that allergic reactions have a basis of psora. The violence of such reactions, occasioned by the release of excessive amounts of histamine, could lead to the conclusion that there is a sycotic process at work in these situations, and it is true that sycosis is a factor in allergy. However, it is necessary to think beyond the initial response and consider why it is happening. The occurrence of an allergic reaction is an abnormal manifestation of immune function. It is a response out of all proportion to the challenge, and indeed the trigger may involve something not normally recognised as a potential allergen.

The author's interpretation is that the key to this is that the response in the allergic situation is an unbalanced response, as also happens with psora in other situations, rather than the more measured deployment of the body's defences that is seen under normal circumstances. The immune system is in effect 'throwing a tantrum', and as with other situations in life this represents a lack of control. There is a failure of the normal direction and control of the immune response, which is essentially a failure of the function of control.

This failure of control function may be part of the inherited miasmatic package of an individual or it may be induced by early abuse of the immature immune system, resulting in permanent damage to its functional integrity. Procedures such as early vaccination and aggressive allopathic or antipathic treatment at an early age may be major factors in the establishment of an allergic state.

The connection of the Tubercular state with allergies is because of the strong psoric component in the make-up of the miasm, coupled with a not inconsiderable sycotic element. The tubercular miasm is characterised by boldness and brashness (Sankaran, 1994), and by the quick change of moods and behaviour (Master, 1992), both of which are exhibited on a physical level in an allergic reaction.

Antipsoric Remedies

Psorinum, the nosode of the psoric miasm, is produced from an infection of the scabies mite, the original material being the discharge from a vesicle. Its remedy picture has certain similarities with that of Sulphur, which Hahnemann regarded as the greatest antipsoric of all, and which he used in his later years to begin the treatment of the majority of his chronic cases, largely on the basis that everyone was inevitably psoric (Handley, 1997) but also because the remedy had the other miasmatic influences well represented. The most marked difference between Psorinum and Sulphur is in the heat modality, where Psorinum greatly desires heat even though conditions are aggravated by it, and Sulphur both dislikes heat and is aggravated by it. Lycopodium and Calcarea Carbonica also have strong antipsoric properties but it must be remembered that they both have significant elements of sycosis also. Whilst Sankaran regards Lycopodium as essentially an antipsoric remedy, he considers it to have a significant antisyphilitic component. Ortega regards both Sulphur and Lycopodium as tending towards a more equimiasmatic balance. As a group the carbon remedies tend to be strongly antipsoric, with survival being an overriding theme of the element. Although many remedies have antipsoric properties to varying extents, Baryta Carbonica, Graphites, Kali Carbonicum, Natrum Carbonicum and Secale should also be considered as major remedies in the group.

CASE 5: *Suppression*

A crossbred tabby cat was six years old at the time of being presented, suffering from severe generalised pruritus. She had been neutered at five months old as a routine but had never received any vaccinations. At one year old she started having epileptic fits for no known reason and was prescribed phenobarbitone and prednisolone, which were continued for four years, with complete control of the convulsions and apparent good health. At this time the skin problems started in a mild form and one month later, after routine investigations, she was diagnosed as diabetic with a very high blood glucose level. Insulin therapy had been started and the steroid stopped, although the phenobarbitone was continued. Linked to regular monitoring the insulin therapy was reduced over a period of three months and finally withdrawn, with clinical normality being maintained apart from the pruritus, which had steadily increased. A blood test one week prior to the homeopathic consultation had shown a normal glucose level. Shortly after the insulin therapy had been introduced she had developed a patch of wet eczema on her neck and an ulcer on her left front leg. These had resolved within about a month with conventional treatment and had not returned.

At the time of the consultation the cat was constantly scratching and had to be kept in a protective collar to prevent self-mutilation. The coat was thin, dry and harsh, but with no scabs, the only lesions being self-inflicted. There was no discolouration or heat in the skin. Conventional treatment of the skin with an oral contraceptive (Ovarid) and anti-histamines had been unsuccessful. Routine systemic flea treatment was being used as a precautionary measure. There were three other cats in the household, none of whom showed any sign of skin problems or flea infestation. The patient was definitely the dominant cat of the four, but only overtly demonstrated her dominance periodically as occasion required. Otherwise she was friendly, with a good appetite and normal thirst. She liked both some heat and some physical petting but retained an independent trait.

Treatment was commenced with Cortisone 30c night and morning for three days, as it was felt that the effects of the conventional steroid therapy were still likely to be present in the system, and that this potential obstacle to cure required removing at the outset. There was a slight initial increase in the degree of irritation following this, but no other material change. This was followed after three weeks by Morgan Bach 30c, selected on the basis of the lack of many definite symptoms apart from the dryness of the coat and the intensity of the pruritis. A dose night and morning for three days was prescribed. However, there was a definite reaction after one tablet, with a complete frenzy developing as a result of the cat's attempts to scratch herself, although the owner was quite clear that it was not a return of the convulsions. The treatment was stopped and the irritation returned to its original state in twelve hours, but did not improve beyond that. However, over the next few days some redness appeared in the skin and the cat became markedly less keen on being near the fire.

On the basis of these changes, Sulphur 30c, three doses in twenty-four hours, was administered. Two weeks later there had been a limited but definite improvement in the skin, and the cat was reported as being happier in herself. A routine blood test showed the glucose level to be normal, as were all other parameters. No further treatment was given and the improvement continued, with the owner being able to remove the collar in another two weeks without risk of a return of the self-mutilation. One month later there was a slight regression that responded to three doses of Sulphur 200c over twenty-four hours and gave complete resolution of the skin symptoms. The owner was able to halve the dose of phenobarbitone without any return of the fits, but, perhaps understandably she could not be persuaded to remove the anticonvulsant entirely. Finally, after a further year without any problems, she was induced to completely remove the medication, which she did without any return of symptoms.

Discussion

Whatever had initiated the convulsions it would appear, in view of the subsequent development of the case, that there was a psoric influence, possibly inherited, which had subsequently been suppressed by the anticonvulsant and steroid treatment. Hence the development of the 'diabetic syndrome' and the wet eczema. It is unclear why a steroid was given as part of the anticonvulsion treatment, but the subsequent events show that its effect was suppressive. All the tissues involved in this disease process have links with the psoric miasm. It should also be noted that the eczema incident was a transitory event – an attempt by the body to exteriorise the disease process. This was unsuccessful due to the treatments being administered and so the disease process became established in a deeper region of the body. As it is suppression of psora that is dominant in this case it is not surprising that an endocrine gland was involved. Activity in both skin and nervous system was being suppressed and the manifestation of disease accordingly moved into another area of psoric influence, namely the homeostatic function of the body. Lifting part of the suppression by the removal of the steroids then allowed the process to be reversed, and the skin became involved in accordance with Hering's Law. Any residual effects of the steroid influence were cleared by using Cortisone 30c.

The presenting picture was undoubtedly psoric with the dry irritant skin and poor hair growth. The lack of a clearer remedy picture at this stage was the reason for the use of the bowel nosode, as a means of producing a more definite picture to prescribe on. There is also a major psoric element in Morgan Bach (Chapter 10), and so the prescription was correct miasmatically. The subsequent appearance of a more definite Sulphur picture as a result enabled the case to be taken forward. Whether the complete removal of the phenobarbitone immediately the irritation had disappeared would have resulted in the reoccurrence of the fits will never be known. However, it is probable that it would not, as the underlying miasmatic imbalance appeared to have been corrected. Hence its continued administration, whilst inevitably having an effect on the body, would not be having any significant suppressive action, and its subsequent successful removal would support that.

CASE 6: *A latent miasm*

A seven-month old entire female St Bernard dog was presented with development problems. Her owners had obtained her at eight weeks of age, having selected her as being the largest in the litter and having what they described as 'a lovely large head'. Their aim was to have the largest dog possible! From the start she had been calm and friendly, but could be lively. Initially she was eating and growing well. She received her first vaccination at ten weeks old with the second injection at twelve weeks, with no obvious immediate reaction to either. She had been wormed by the breeder at six weeks of age, using a standard commercial preparation, and again at the time of vaccination, on that occasion using a prescription-only medicine (Drontal Plus).

From around four months of age she had become progressively slower and her appetite decreased to the point where she had to be hand fed. She would no longer play or voluntarily go for a walk, although she still liked to be petted. She would markedly seek heat and lie near a source for as long as allowed. Her thirst was unchanged. There was no vomiting or diarrhoea. Although her skeleton had continued to grow, the rate had slowed and there was a poor covering of flesh over the whole body. The head was still noticeable for its size in relation to the rest of the body. She was 'cow-hocked', with both hocks (ankles) turning inwards, and the feet pointing outwards. Both front legs showed extreme dropping of the carpus (wrist) to the extent that the posterior surfaces of the lower legs were in contact with the ground. Both legs were also turning outward from the carpus. There was no excessive thickening around the joints and no pain on palpation or movement.

The original veterinary surgeon had diagnosed a 'nutritional deficiency and imbalance caused by an unknown metabolic disorder'. Mineral and vitamin supplements together with anabolic steroids had produced no improvement. An orthopaedic specialist had diagnosed 'irreversible tendon and ligament weakness with possible growth plate insufficiency', and advised joint fixation. Although the skeleton appeared large and solid, radiography had revealed a thin cortex in the long bones of the limbs. It was at this point that homeopathic treatment was sought.

A blood sample was taken for both routine screening and in-depth thyroid investigation. No significant abnormalities were found in the haematology and other standard parameters. Treatment commenced with a nosode prepared from the standard canine vaccine, with 30c night and morning for three days being administered. This was selected on an aetiological basis, as the onset of symptoms so soon after vaccination was considered significant. This was followed by Calc. Carb. 30c, three doses in twenty-four hours, as probably being the correct constitutional prescription, in view of the temperament and the fundamental size and proportion of the body; the great desire for heat and the unwillingness to move were also considerations.

Two weeks later the dog was eating well again and was livelier. A marked improvement in the appetite had occurred by the end of the course of nosode. There was no material change in the legs. Calcarea Fluorica 30c was prescribed once daily for two weeks. It was felt that while there was undoubtedly a strong element of a Calcium remedy in the constitution, another remedy from that group with potentially a more particular effect on the tissues of the limbs would be advantageous. A week later the laboratory report confirmed an allergic thyroiditis, probably due to vaccination. A further three weeks had the dog back to her old self as far as appetite and temperament were concerned. The hind legs now appeared normal and the carpi on the front were no longer rubbing on the ground. Calc. Fluor. was continued for a further week at the same dose. A month later there had been a 50% improvement in the carriage of the front legs, but progress had ceased. Mobility was now improved, but there appeared to be some pain in her limbs as she would not rest in one position for long after moving about. The prescription was changed to Ruta 30c because of the restlessness and also because of the particular affinity of the remedy for ligaments and tendons. It was given night and morning for ten days. The discomfort disappeared and the improvement continued without further treatment. She finally developed into the dog that the owners had always hoped for.

Discussion

Although this condition was triggered by vaccination, the major upset was psoric rather than the sycosis commonly associated with classic vaccinosis. Vaccination can produce an allergic reaction in the thyroid, and allergy is principally a psoric reaction. Although there was undoubtedly sycosis present from the challenge, this was secondary to psora in the clinical picture of slowness, lack of reactiveness, and failure to thrive. In view of the severity of the clinical reaction in this case, it is likely that there was a latent psora in the patient's hereditary make-up, which was brought into life by the challenge. The timing of the onset in relation to the vaccination was felt to be too much of a coincidence, and the nosode was given on the basis of 'never well since'. Although there had been no observed reaction to either of the vaccination injections, this is never a guarantee that some damage has not been done. Compton Burnett considered in relation to smallpox vaccination that the worst cases of vaccinosis occurred where there had been no appearance of a local skin reaction at the site of inoculation (*Vaccinosis and its Cure by Thuja*). This was considered by the conventional world to have indicated a failure of the vaccine to have stimulated an immunity, and the procedure was usually repeated until such a reaction was obtained. Homeopathically, of course, a very different interpretation is given, with the absence of a skin reaction indicating a failure by the body to throw the challenge outward in any way.

The presenting picture indicated an antipsoric remedy that nevertheless has a significant sycotic element. Hence the use of Calc. Carb. in addition to the nosode. Following these remedies the picture changed, with the psoric manifestations becoming less but not disappearing. Calc. Fluor. was prescribed on the basis of its constitutional connection and its tissue affinity for ligaments, the choice being reflected in the miasmatic make-up of the remedy, exhibiting the sycotic trait of new tissue growth and syphilitic component of destruction.

Once the aetiological aspect of the case had been cleared, the presenting psoric picture was then addressed. As this yielded to treatment the more sycotic aspects could be given more prominence in remedy selection, although psora always remained a factor.

CASE 7: *An inherited miasm*

A fourteen-year-old girl, suffered with an erythematous rash on her face, neck, arms, and hands. This had first appeared some eighteen months previously, shortly after the onset of her periods. Although not constantly present, the only time when the skin was clear was for about one week while after the end of a period. The rash would begin to reappear about a week before the onset of the next period, build to a peak during it, and settle some three to four days after its end. The periods were on a regular four-weekly cycle and were described as moderate. The rash was essentially non-irritant except for certain times in bed. She had no difficulty going to sleep but would sometimes wake with a desire to scratch. The warmth of a room did not affect the situation, although there was no great liking for heat. She was, however, happy to be outside in most weather conditions. Various creams and ointments, plus antihistamine tablets had been tried without success before turning to homeopathy.

She also suffered from hay fever, and her skin was generally sensitive to a range of detergents and soaps. Exposure would result in the appearance of the rash on any part of the body. Some of the topical treatments had aggravated her face and arms but no accurate record had been kept of which they were. Her hay fever occurred every year for the 'whole season', the severity and duration being related to the pollen count. Antihistamines had produced only limited success in relieving the condition.

The usual childhood vaccinations had been given with no apparent ill-effects. She had suffered a bad attack of chickenpox at the age of seven, but her medical history was otherwise unremarkable.

There was a history of hay fever and skin problems on both sides of her family. A maternal aunt had suffered with acne for many years, and her father and his sister also continued to be affected into adult life. Her mother would have attacks of what had been described as 'nervous asthma' at times of stress.

She was an only child, described as a friendly, outgoing and affectionate girl, her only real limitation being an acute sensitivity about the rash. There were no pets in the household. Her appetite was described as normal and her thirst as small. Her only real dislike was of the skin on custard or milk. She would not drink warm milk, but would if it was cold straight from the fridge. She liked sweets and chocolate but did not eat them because they made her skin worse. She had no major fears, her main worry being that her skin would never clear. She dreamt a lot but not about anything in particular, although she described most of her dreams as being sad.

Treatment was begun initially with a prescription of Pulsatilla 200c night and morning for three days. This appeared to fit the friendly and easygoing temperament, together with the general symptoms of dislike of heat, enjoyment of being outside, thirstlessness, and the appearance of the rash. There was also the aetiology of the onset at puberty and the continuing link to the sexual cycle. The course was administered after one of her periods, whilst the skin was clear. The skin erupted as previously but it was felt that it was 'not quite as bad as usual'.

The remedy was repeated at 200c night and morning for two days during the next clear time. This resulted in the rash not appearing until the period actually started although its intensity was as great as ever. The next period was allowed to pass without further treatment and the same pattern of non-appearance until the period showed was seen. Doses of Pulsatilla 200c and 1M at the subsequent periods produced only a slight further reduction in the intensity of the skin problem.

Because of the strong family history of allergic reactions, together with the clear allergic tendencies, the prescription was then changed to Tuberculinum Bovinum 200c night and morning for three days. This resulted in a marked reduction in the skin's intensity at the next eruption, and this was maintained through the next two periods without further treatment, although there was still some eruption. Pulsatilla 1M, three doses in twenty-four hours was then given. The subsequent period was very much heavier than expected and the skin eruption virtually non existent. Following that, the periods then reverted to their normal intensity and the skin has remained essentially clear since then, with a corresponding reduction in the general sensitivity to detergents and other common household products.

Treatment had been begun in October and continued over the winter months. The hay fever in the following summer was much milder than anticipated in spite of a high pollen count at times.

Discussion

The family history was obviously of great significance in this case, with the inheritance of strong and similar traits from both sides of her family tree. However, whilst psora was undoubtedly a factor, the initial presentation of a condition linked to reproductive function, together with the timing of onset around puberty and the presenting picture of the patient as an easygoing and friendly girl, indicated the use of the sycotic-based Pulsatilla as the starting point. The manifestation of the condition as apparently a skin problem might have led to the assumption that it was essentially psoric. However, the strong allergic aspects of both the case and the family histories pointed to the involvement of the tubercular miasm, with its strong connection to allergic reactions, as the underlying influence. Hence the use of the nosode when the action of the Pulsatilla appeared to be exhausted. It is significant that this gave an improvement in the other allergic conditions manifesting in the patient, but also that it was necessary to return to Pulsatilla in order to complete the resolution of the presenting complaint. The change in the intensity of the period under its influence would indicate that there was still some sycotic action that needed to be cleared before final resolution could occur. It is worth noting that there is also a significant psoric element in Pulsatilla, which fits in with the overall direction of the case. It is also interesting to note that a severe attack of chickenpox in childhood had not removed the miasmatic imbalance, possibly because the underlying imbalance was due to the presence of an established mixed miasm that had been inherited from both sides of her family.

Chapter 8

Sycosis

Basic Concepts

Hahnemann regarded sycosis as clinically the least important of the three miasms. His opening remarks on sycosis in *Chronic Diseases* state: '… sycosis, as being that miasma which has produced by far the fewest chronic diseases, and has only been dominant from time to time.' It is possible this opinion may have been influenced by the fact that, whilst it can cause fatalities, conventionally gonorrhoea is the least serious of the venereal diseases, generally without the life-threatening aspect of syphilis. Also, in spite of a number of surges in incidence, usually linked to the activities of armies, its incidence showed a reducing pattern from its peak in the early years of the nineteenth century. Hahnemann cites the years 1809–1814 as being the height of its spread, with steady decline after that (at least up to 1828). But even if Hahnemann's assessment was true in his time it is doubtful whether it is still true today. Many of the disease patterns, notably cancer, calculi and female reproductive problems, encountered in modern medicine have a major sycotic component, and many modern treatments and preventive procedures seem predisposed towards the establishment of the miasm. This is especially, but not exclusively, true in the reproductive sphere, and it is here that the effects of suppressive procedures are often seen at their worst.

As with psora, the name is derived from one of the major clinical features of the miasm. The Greek words *sukon* (a fig) and *osis* (forming), combine to describe the process and the particular type of warts that are characteristic of the picture. But, as with psora, the name does little to describe the full nature and extent of the reactions that are induced in the body by the miasm.

Equally misleading from the homeopathic point of view is the close connection that was made in the early days between sycosis and the gonorrhoeal infection. There was much diagnostic confusion with syphilis, with many doctors believing that the two were in fact only one disease. John Hunter (1728–1793) at one time took this view, but

Hahnemann always considered them as two separate entities. In *Chronic Diseases* he states '[gonorrhoea] was treated almost always in an inefficient and injurious manner, internally with mercury, because it was considered homogeneous with the venereal chancre disease [syphilis].' Thus in spite of its decline the infection was still a major clinical entity in Hahnemann's day, and it has many features of the typical sycotic disease. The saying 'Gonorrhoea is the forerunner of catarrh' hints at the way that the infection can both establish and activate the sycotic tendency. However, in spite of the superficial connection there is much more to the miasm than just the particular venereal disease and its suppression. Not every case of gonorrhoea will produce the typical figwarts, and the symptoms of the disease by no means represent the full picture of sycosis.

Clinical Manifestations

Sycosis may be considered to equate to the hydrogenoid constitution of Grauvogl. As the name implies, water, and reactions to water, are major considerations in this type. There is a tendency to retain water in the tissues, and externally there is a marked sensitivity of all symptoms to humidity, cold and damp. Symptoms are often aggravated whenever there is a change of weather.

Sycosis is associated with excesses of all kinds and produces those conditions that often are described as 'hyper'. There is overreaction, exaggeration, and a general lack of moderation on both the mental and physical levels. Mentally, the miasm produces extremes of both behaviour and tastes, and paradoxical opposites may be seen in the same patient, with marked mood swings. The tendency, however, is often towards the more antisocial forms of behaviour. The shifting of symptoms from one side of the body to the other is a reflection on the physical level of the mood swings that are seen in the mental sphere. A definite modality of conditions being worse from sunrise to sunset is seen, while there may be a marked amelioration around midnight when the protective mental mask found in the miasm is dropped. However, some symptoms, noticeably headaches, are worse at night. In general, symptoms are better for pressure, and lying on the abdomen gives relief in many conditions. As would be expected there is a marked mental reaction when any external influence goes to extremes, and the sycotic type is worse for storms and related upsets. Similarly, strong physical stimuli generally will produce marked adverse reactions.

Pathological discharges bring relief. As indicated above, this is the miasm of irritation of mucous surfaces and the production of catarrh. These discharges are usually green or yellow in colour, with much congestion of the associated mucous membranes. The discharges are strong-smelling, often fishy, and will stain materials with which they come into contact with a yellowish hue. The perspiration has a sweet smell to it and is usually copious.

The irritation of the mucous membranes that produces the typical discharges is also mirrored in the mental sphere. Much anger is seen in the type, which may be provoked by the slightest upset or accident, and often by pain, which can easily become extreme. Even a worsening of the weather may provoke a bout of fury. There is also a theme of 'covering up' in the sycotic picture, with a delusion that they are vulnerable and will break easily. They do not trust even themselves completely, and the covering up is essentially a survival mechanism, with fixed ideas and routines providing a perceived degree of security. This will manifest on the mental plane as a constant checking and rechecking of what they have done in order to avoid both change and mistakes. They are constantly suspicious and jealous, and have a desire to protect themselves by hiding what they perceive as their true, unworthy nature, or their one dark guilty secret. This desire tends to make them devious. In extreme cases the feelings of unworthiness will lead to suicide, which is usually premeditated.

There are feelings of being a split personality, which are often suppressed in order to control the insecurity that such a state implies, and to appear 'normal'. The desire to appear normal may manifest itself in packs or herds as those animals who always remain in the middle of the group, never pushing themselves to the front, nor falling behind. They will copy the behaviour of others, and these are the dogs who will always bark if another dog starts. Similarly people will tend to follow the accepted social norms or always copy the behaviour of their peer group. Alternatively the type may hide behind a great show of ostentation, or, believing that 'attack is the best form of defence', may become domineering to the point of cruelty. These feelings also lead to dreams and delusions of physical separation, and to a restlessness linked to dissatisfaction rather than to the anxiety of psora. The sycotic patient is selfish and irritable with fixed ideas and opinions, but, within those limits, extremely practical and efficient. There is a desire to hurry through everything. Movements are hurried and time seems to pass too slowly, indeed there may be a general derangement of the time sense.

The theme of covering up is seen physically in the form of a general thickening of tissues and the formation of exostoses. This has the effect of fixing tissues and organs and leading to restriction of movement and function. Arthritis and rheumatism are commonly linked to the miasm, and these are painful.

Paradoxically, many sycotic conditions are slow and insidious in onset, although once established they may contain an 'explosive' element (e.g. diarrhoea).This characteristic is often seen in birds, where conditions come on undetected until the sudden appearance of some violent symptomatology. As onset is often slow, so recovery is often gradual. In many cases where there is more than one miasm manifesting, it will be the sycotic that is the most prominent. Sycosis produces many painful conditions with much spasm, the pains being generally relieved by motion and pressure. The alimentary system produces many painful symptoms due to spasm. Colic and many diarrhoeas are sycotic, the latter often having a urgency due to increased peristaltic motion. Diarrhoea is accompanied by straining, which may lead to rectal prolapse, and the stools are offensive, sour, and tending towards a green colour. The fishy smell that is typically sycotic is frequently met with in the motion, and there is often a fishy taste in the mouth. There is usually a desire for meat, which is easily converted into uric acid. Rich foods, alcohol and salt are also desired.

There can be a wide range of aversions and aggravations linked to food, an extreme example being the unusual symptom of a carnivore who has the general or local modality of being < meat. The type tends to eat quickly, but this produces feelings of fullness. These are the animals (usually carnivores) who will eat so quickly that they induce vomiting, and too high an intake of water at one time can produce abdominal symptoms. There may be slow digestion and absorption from the alimentary tract. Appendicitis is essentially a sycotic condition, with the underlying irritation and overproduction from a mucous surface (Chapter 2).

The hyperplastic tendency leads to the formation of calculi and deposits of all kinds in the tissues. Bladder, kidney, gall-bladder and salivary calculi are all part of the sycotic diathesis. Similarly, the accumulation of uric acid in the tissues as is seen in gout is a sycotic manifestation. Wounds that heal with the production of surplus external tissue (proud flesh) do so under the sycotic influence. Excess scar tissue associated with healing is also seen. Throughout the body benign tumours, polyps and warts are found.

The skin and extremities of the body manifest many signs of the sycotic influence. Nails, claws and hooves are often affected. This may show as thickening of the tissues, with ridges often being felt. At the same time the quality of the horn may be poor due to its too rapid growth. The skin will show a range of warts, cysts and benign lumps; there is often increased pigmentation, which may be excessive and accompanied by marked thickening of the tissues. Hair loss and pigmentation in circular lesions are often seen. The changes in the skin may cause the patient no bother at all, but severe irritation is also seen. When eruptions and pruritis are present they may be aggravated by eating meat. The skin tends to be greasy, and this will be felt in the coats of animals rather than the dry or silky feel that is normal. Conditions of the ears, often accompanied by painful ulcerations and offensive fishy discharges, are a feature of the miasm.

Cardiac hypertrophy and functional irregularities are seen, with sudden, sharp pains. Tachycardia occurs and the pulse is often weak.

Oedema and discharges from the mucous surfaces are characteristic of the respiratory system. The mucus may block the nasal passages, and if it is deep in the system expectoration is difficult. Breathing is often rapid.

The urinary and genital systems are major seats of sycotic activity. There is cystitis with straining and painful micturition. Recurrent cystitis will lead to thickening of the bladder wall. Hypertrophy and inflammation of the prostate are features, along with a general tendency to inflammation in the genital system. Increased libido in both sexes and low fertility in females is seen. Breast and uterine pains during menses are common. Endometritis and inflammatory pelvic disease are sycotic in origin.

Suppression and the Reproductive System

Suppression figures as largely in the aetiology of sycosis as in the other miasms. The confusion of gonorrhoea with syphilis in the early days led to much treatment with mercury in material doses, which was therapeutically ineffective and did nothing but harm. Equally harmful, and arguably more so, was the practice of cauterising the skin lesions or the use of various ointments on them. Although from the conventional perspective the removal of the external lesions appeared to be a desirable thing, homeopathically this represented a major suppression of the body's attempt to cure the condition.

Suppression of the established miasm can drive the disease process into any part of the body, but predominantly into the urino-genital system. The link between sycosis and the reproductive faculty is the strongest example of the affinity of a particular miasm for a specific body system, and the close physical link between the urinary and genital systems results in both being involved in sycotic reactions. The need to reproduce is one of the most basic functions in all species, and in the context of the survival of any species it is the most important. Consequently, on a physiological level, the creation of new tissues within the system designed to carry out this role can be regarded as the most important basic function of all. Philosophically, the reproductive system may be regarded as the 'spiritual home' of the physiological sycotic function. The syphilitic miasm also has some connections to the reproductive system, and the combination of these two often results in the development of the most life-threatening of conditions.

Suppression is generally thought of as being concerned solely with disease states, but it must always be remembered that the inhibition of any normal type of function is also a form of suppression, capable of creating a miasm in exactly the same way as interference with a disease process can. This aspect – the inhibition of normal physiological function – has attained a much greater prominence in the modern age, and is one of the reasons for the big increase in the sycotic miasm as a clinical entity. Much of this inhibition is of the normal reproductive functions, either by chemical or surgical means, with a corresponding effect on sycotic manifestations. Chemical contraception is a major cause of sycosis, especially, for the reasons discussed above, within the reproductive system. However, the effects of suppression are not confirmed to the reproductive system. It can be argued that the clinical manifestations of sycosis now form the major part of the most common condition seen, and that in a sense sycosis may now be considered to be the most important of the three miasms. (It is instructive to reflect on the change in the balance of the miasms since Hahnemann's time. He considered that the clinical pictures he encountered were overwhelmingly manifestations of the predominant psoric miasm, with sycosis being the least influential. Today there is a better understanding of the histopathology behind clinical syndromes. In addition, there have been enormous changes in medical treatments and physiological interventions since Hahnemann's time. This has resulted in a significant shift in the miasmatic balance of current clinical syndromes, and these insights can be of practical use in treatment.)

Vaccination and Sycosis

The other area in which sycosis is a major factor, and which has contributed in no small part to the increase in its manifestation, is vaccination. Whatever the other considerations in the whole vaccine picture, the miasmatic aspects of the procedure must be recognised and addressed if major difficulties are to be avoided.

Many of the physiological processes set in motion by challenge of an infective or invasive nature involve the immune system in general, and the reticuloendothelial system in particular. The sycotic state has been described by French authors (Bernard, 1950; Fortier-Bernovillie, 1934) as one of chronic reticuloendotheliosis, which they equate with a premature ageing of the immune system. In view of the systems of the body that are involved in the creation of immunity by vaccination, it is not surprising that in miasmatic terms the consequences should be predominantly sycotic. However, the two other miasmatic influences may on occasion manifest as a result of vaccination, and must be recognised as such. The hypoglycaemic state that may be induced is in fact secondary to a typically sycotic hyperinsulinaemia, while the allergic thyroiditis associated with the procedure has a major psoric component and may result in a typically psoric hypothyroid state. The haemorrhagic and demyelination states seen in some post-vaccination cases are predominantly syphilitic.

It is not appropriate to explore the full vaccine story in this context, and the reader is referred to Burnett, *Vaccinosis and its Cure by Thuja* (1897) and Saxton and Gregory, *Textbook of Veterinary Homeopathy* (2005) for consideration of the broader issues. However, two aspects are particularly relevant to miasms, irrespective of species.

Firstly, the route of most vaccination bypasses the natural route of infection and this produces a shock to the systemic part of the immune system, particularly the reticuloendothelial system. Since most vaccination is carried out on young immature subjects of all species, this shock can have long-term consequences. Infection via the natural route activates the cellular immune response, which thus alerts the rest of the system to the coming challenge. But in a natural infection this local cellular response would involve the production of discharges from the mucous surfaces as part of the disease process. The failure to involve the local tissues in the immune response, and hence to generate the local discharges, can be regarded as a form of suppression. A body undergoing vaccination experiences the simulation of a disease without at the same time being allowed the natural working-through of the means of coping with that disease. In practical terms there is no difference between this and the forcible removal of a disease manifestation, as discussed before. Vaccines that do follow the natural route may still be capable of creating the same upset to the body (these are more commonly found in the veterinary sphere, although the human oral polio vaccine was one such). The attenuation of the disease-producing agent can result in a failure to stimulate the local tissues to the necessary degree, although the size of the dose may still be strong enough to have some systemic effect. This effect, as discussed above, will not be the same as a normal balanced reaction.

Secondly, if the body finds an alternative route by which to eliminate the disease, and this is blocked by inappropriate treatment, then problems will also arise. Any treatment, either local or systemic, of the desirable natural discharges via the natural route will be suppressive in its effect (see Case 8, facing). Either vaccination itself, or the suppression of the body's attempts to deal with it, can lead to the condition homeopaths recognise as vaccinosis (Saxton, 2005). As shown above, the direct effect of vaccination is an inflammatory reaction within the immune system, which is primarily sycotic, although the exact symptom picture in individual cases may be affected by the influence of other, usually inherited, miasmatic traits.

Antisycotic Remedies

Medorrhinum is the nosode of the sycotic miasm. It is prepared from the urethral discharge of a patient suffering from gonorrhoea.

The other well known antisycotic remedy is undoubtedly Thuja. As a result of Burnett's work it is often thought of as *the only* vaccinosis remedy. Although it is certainly a major vaccinosis remedy, it is incorrect to consider it as the only one. A marked feature of Thuja is heavy pigmentation and thickening of the skin, and in animals enlargement of the nipples, even in those subjects that have been surgically neutered. It is not, however, the only major antisycotic remedy, and it has many indications outside the vaccinosis situation. Similarly, other antisycotic remedies have uses in connection with vaccination (as has Sulphur). Among other remedies to be considered in sycotic situations are Antimonium Tartaricum, Kali Sulphuricum, Malandrinum, Mezereum, Natrum Muriaticum, Natrum Sulphuricum, Pulsatilla, Sabina, Sepia, Staphysagria, Silica and Triticum Repens. Because of their origin from within the reproductive system, the Lac remedies all have strong sycotic features. Although other miasms are markedly present in the pictures of Argentum Nitricum and Nitric Acid, both remedies have significant sycotic elements.

CASE 8: *The genital connection*

A four-year-old entire male Borzoi dog (sometimes known as the Russian Greyhound) was presented with a history of recurrent attacks of prostatitis over the previous two years. There had been six attacks in all, with three of them occurring in the previous five months. The first three attacks had been more evenly spaced over the previous nineteen months. All had been treated with antibiotics and steroids and had apparently settled easily. During the attacks there was loss of appetite and thirst, great depression, slight ineffectual rectal straining and the passage of apparently normal urine in a slow stream. There was no history of illness of any kind and no indication as to why the attacks had started. The only veterinary attention had been for annual booster vaccinations, but the dates of these were unknown. On one of these occasions mention had been made of a discharge from the sheath, which was considered to be of no clinical consequence as far as the dog was concerned and was only mentioned because of its perceived hygienic implications. Unfortunately no accurate description of the discharge could be obtained. A course of antibiotics had been prescribed, to no effect, after which the discharge had been ignored and finally disappeared of its own accord.

The owner, while being pleasant and eager to help, was unused to both dogs and the homeopathic method. Help was being sought not out of conviction, but because the conventional approach was not giving permanent relief and the overall situation was worsening. Consequently the information yielded by the consultation was minimal. The owner 'liked the breed' and hence a puppy had been acquired, but he essentially knew nothing about them. All questions about temperament, desires, aversions and modalities received the same answer of 'just like a normal dog'!

The latest attack was just settling after the usual course of conventional treatment, and there was still slight depression with a poor appetite present. The dog walked and stood with a definite arch to the back. Rectal temperature was normal. Clinical examination revealed an enlarged, soft prostate, which was slightly tender on palpation, but no other abnormality.

The only reliable observable symptom available, apart from some extremely common ones linked to general malaise, was the continuing enlargement of the prostate and the associated tenderness, although even with this the effects of treatment had to be borne in mind. The reported slow passage of urine was considered to be of some significance, as in the dog the proximity of the prostate to the rectum means that the usual consequence of an enlarged prostate is an interference with rectal rather than with bladder function. The history of a discharge from the sheath was considered, together with the fact that it had not apparently returned during any of the attacks. The location of the presenting complaint was also taken into account. Accordingly, Medorrhinum 30c, three doses in twenty-four hours, was given. The next day the dog was behaving in a depressed manner again and the appetite had once more disappeared completely. After a further twenty-four hours the dog was drinking a little but was still depressed. A thick, yellow odourless discharge had appeared from the sheath. No further treatment was given. Three days later the appetite was improving and more interest was being shown in life generally. The discharge was now copious but changing to a paler, thinner consistency.

Ten days later all was back to normal, with no discharge and no prostatic enlargement palpable. Re-examination eighteen months later for a lameness problem confirmed that there had been no recurrence.

Discussion

The essence of this case could have applied to any species. The somewhat limited amount of information obtained from the consultation was unusual, even by veterinary standards, and the information that was available was largely of such a common nature as to be of limited help in prescribing. Consideration of what could be gleaned, or inferred, produced possible rubrics such as:

Prostate Gland; pain
Prostate Gland; swelling
Prostate Gland; inflammation
Abdomen; pain; bending; double; ameliorates
Urethra; discharges (?Gleety)

This did not yield much that was of help with individualising the case, the rubrics being somewhat general as far as a strict repertorising approach was concerned.

However, consideration of the location of the problem, together with such information as was available, gave a way into the heart of the problem. The condition, in spite of repeated suppression, was still remaining within the same system, with no evidence of any deepening of the disease process. The fact that it was the reproductive system that was involved provided a strong indication of a sycotic connection, and the history of a discharge and the nature of the lesion, involving enlargement of the prostate, confirmed the diagnosis on a miasmatic level. The miasmatic connection, plus such symptoms as were available, was strong enough to indicate the initial use of the miasmatic nosode rather than any other remedy, although the major remedies indicated by (retrospective) repertorisation have strong antisycotic features. Use of these (Staphysagria, Pulsatilla) would possibly have had some beneficial effect, but would probably not have produced the direct cure that was obtained. There were, in fact, no further prostatic troubles and the dog died some six years later, never having had any major health problems after his treatment as above, in spite of continuing with annual booster vaccinations. The presumed cause of death was heart failure, but no post-mortem was carried out.

CASE 9: *The predominant miasm*

An entire German Shepherd Dog was two and a half years old at the time of his first presentation. He was a large example of the breed in respect of his skeletal development, but his lack of weight in relation to his size was a cause of concern (35 kg against an estimated normal of 40–45 kg). He had been chosen at seven weeks of age because he had been the largest in the litter. The main presenting complaint was a marked generalised pruritis that had been present to some degree since he was six months old. No lesions were visible on the skin, which was dry. The hair was thin in places, mainly those areas that could be most vigorously attacked by teeth or claws, but there were no bald areas. There was no clear time modality to the scratching. The dog liked a certain amount of heat but could become too warm, when he would move away from the source and not return. He was happy to be out in the sun if he was active, but would not lie in it.

His appetite was poor and capricious. A wide selection of commercial foods, both tinned and dry, had been tried – he would eat a new flavour enthusiastically for a few days and then lose interest.

His life was lived, as the owner described it, 'at the double', with walks being his greatest pleasure. Although he settled well during the consultation he was alert to the slightest sound. He liked company but not cuddles.

He had received his first vaccination at eight weeks of age. Seven days later he had been taken back to the vet with vomiting, loss of appetite and urinary frequency with blood in the urine. A course of antibiotics had been given and he had apparently recovered, although his appetite became poor from that time on. He subsequently received his second vaccination at twelve weeks old without further incident.

He had started to scratch when he was around six months old, for no apparent reason, and a thick preputial discharge had appeared. Skin investigations had revealed no mites or fungal infections. Treatment with antihistamines and steroids controlled the problem but did not cure, and occasional injections and oral courses of steroids had been administered as appeared necessary. The preputial discharge remained to some degree at all times. After five months the urinary problem returned and was again treated with antibiotics. A booster vaccination at fifteen months old resulted in an increase in the skin irritation and an attack of colitis. The colitis had been resolved with Salazopyrin but the skin worsened steadily from that time. After two months a lump appeared on the left pinna; it was surgically removed and shown to be a lipoma. One month later there was an attack of what was described as 'polyarthritis' and another lump appeared on the right side of the neck, which was again removed. The scratching was still bad, and as further skin tests revealed nothing he was referred for homeopathy.

Treatment was begun with Thuja 30c night and morning for three days, because of the strong connection in the history to vaccination. The timing of the initial reaction at nine weeks old and the essentially sycotic nature of the subsequent symptomatology dictated the remedy choice. Three weeks later the owner reported a marked reduction of 50% in the scratching, which had occurred after about a week, and was being maintained. The discharge from the sheath was reducing. During the second week there had been two days when the motions, although normal, had been covered in mucus. Thuja 200c was repeated for two days night and morning. This did not produce any significant reduction in the pruritis, but some patches of redness appeared on the skin, although there was no heat accompanying them. The appetite improved somewhat and there was more mucus on the motions. Most of the scratching was now on the legs rather than the body. Sulphur 200c night and morning for three days was prescribed, as fitting the changed presenting skin picture more closely, and as having a broader based miasmatic balance than the Thuja. All scratching ceased within one week, but returned after ten days. The discharge from the sheath was still present and unchanged in nature but further reducing in quantity, and the mucus had returned to some degree in the motions.

Because the action of the Thuja appeared to be blocked in spite of the symptom picture still being predominantly sycotic, three doses of Sycotic Co. 30c were administered over twenty-four hours. This approach follows the recognised rationale for using a bowel nosode to reactivate the effectiveness of an associated remedy. All scratching ceased for two weeks and then returned, but only on the feet. The discharge from the sheath was unchanged. Another three doses of Thuja 200c in twenty-four hours were then administered. This produced an increase of all symptoms for a week after which everything cleared for five weeks. After that time there was a return of the irritation on the front legs with no lesions. Sulphur 200c night and morning for two days was administered and the irritation ceased. After three years the dog is still free of all symptoms and is bright and lively. He continues to live life at speed and with great enthusiasm. His appetite has improved and is now adequate. His weight is now within the normal range, but remains at the lower end of that range. In view of his lifestyle, that is not considered surprising.

Discussion

A presenting complaint involving the skin is commonly found in both human and animal practice. The initial reaction here could have been that the problem was basically psoric, with a dry skin showing no lesions. However, while there was undoubtedly some psora, the history clearly shows a sycotic tendency running throughout, with the urinary involvement, the mucoid colitis, the preputial discharge and the lipomas on the ear and neck. The initial reaction to the vaccination represented the body's attempt to clear itself of the effects of the vaccine. The presumption of a urinary infection and the use of antibiotics resulted in a suppression of that attempt, with the subsequent appearance of symptoms elsewhere. The eruption of a lipoma following steroid treatment and a booster vaccination was indicative of a further suppressive situation, and the flaring of a new syndrome plus the subsequent growth of another lipoma after removal confirmed it.

The predominance of the sycosis dictated that the starting point must be a major sycotic remedy, and given the aetiology of vaccination and the overall symptom picture, Thuja was selected. This produced some improvement, but the control of the sycotic dominance allowed the psoric influence to increase. Hence the prescriptions of Thuja, after initial success, failed to make further progress in the case. Sulphur, as a more miasmatically equal remedy, addressed the new miasmatic balance as it presented. The Sycotic Co., with its connection to sycosis, was given because of the perceived continuing presence of the sycotic miasm, and the subsequent reaction following a return to Thuja confirmed that. The final treatment involved the psoric miasm before complete balance was restored. It is interesting to note in this case the working of Hering's Law alongside the miasmatic changes.

CASE 10: *A mixed but clear pattern*

A 41-year-old single lady sought help because of a prolonged spell of indeterminate ill health. She was a senior veterinary practice nurse who very much enjoyed her job and described herself as 'doing it well'. Her employers agreed with this assessment.

She had received the normal childhood vaccinations. An attack of nephritis when she was fifteen years old, lasting two weeks, was the only illness she could recall other than an episode of food poisoning sometime during her teens. She was an only child of strict parents, and still felt bitter about the restrictive nature of her upbringing when, in her own words, 'her parents didn't like the idea of her growing up'. Her father had been a workaholic with rigid attitudes who had died of cancer. She had always felt great difficulty in getting emotionally close to him, and consequently as a teenager she had undertaken activities (mechanics and restoring cars) that he, rather than she, was interested in. She described her mother as a 'control freak', but in spite of that had remained close to her until her death from natural causes.

Some two years prior to the homeopathic consultation, she had developed what had been diagnosed as irritable bowel syndrome linked to anxiety and stress. During attacks she had urgency and abdominal pains. The motions contained mucus but no blood, and were passed without excessive straining. She had declined conventional treatment and was taking herbs under the direction of a qualified herbal practitioner. These were providing control of the problem, but it returned when she stopped the medication.

Six months previously she had began passing blood in her urine, and was feeling constantly tired. Urine had been passed normally and without pain. Investigations by her doctor had revealed leucocytes, nitrites and protein in the urine in addition to the blood. Haematology tests revealed an elevated creatinine level, which had returned to normal in later samples. The conventional diagnosis had been a kidney infection, and several courses of various antibiotics had been given without benefit to the overall condition, whilst the bowel symptoms were intensified. She had returned to just the herbal treatment, with additions to the prescription in view of the conventional diagnosis. A check just prior to the homeopathic consultation had shown that the leucocytes and nitrites had gone from the urine but the blood and protein remained at moderate levels (++ on a screening dipstick scale of 1–4) while a blood test had revealed a moderate anaemia but no other abnormalities. Appetite was unaffected. There had been no increase in thirst since the troubles began, but that had always been large, and she had always wanted a long drink first thing in the morning. She had never been keen on alcohol, basically restricting her drinking to social events. Since the onset of the irritable bowels she had stopped drinking alcohol completely as she felt that it aggravated the condition. There had been no enlargement of the external lymph nodes at any stage. Her motions were now always on the soft side with occasional attack of colitis as above, but without flatulence. It was a great effort for her to do her job and she felt absolutely exhausted at the end of each day. She had always slept well, and continued to do so as far as the length of time she was asleep, but she was now awakening tired. She was aware of dreaming regularly but usually could not remember the content of them.

Over the years she had used various forms of the contraceptive pill, but all had given problems (unspecified) and it was some four years since their last use. Periods were described as 'now being normal'.

Her own assessment of herself was that she had some mental rigidity and intolerance. She described herself as shy, and although sympathetic to others disliked receiving similar care. She preferred all aspects of life to be structured and organised, and her top priority was always to avoid 'erosion of her personal space'. She was obsessive about the accuracy of the written word. She liked to be tidy but hoarded everything, and so generally didn't achieve her aim. She consequently had periodic blitzes of cleaning and tidying. She was conscientious but not obsessive about the cleanliness of the practice theatre and ward. Every situation and happening was intellectually rationalised. She disliked cold food and strongly objected to anything slimy, otherwise she would eat most things. She disliked the cold but became listless in very hot weather. She would not of choice go out in even light rain, but had no strong feelings about thunder.

Various remedies, such as Arsenicum Album, Carcinosin, Natrum Muriaticum and Sepia suggest themselves as of a result of the presenting features of the case, such as a degree of intolerance, the dislike of consolation, the weight loss, blood in urine, exhaustion, tidy instinct, aggravation from alcohol and dislike of cold. The family history and the general mental state of the overwhelming desire for privacy pointed towards Natrum Muriaticum. Although there was a control element in childhood there was not the performance requirement that is often present in Carcinosin, and the miasmatic picture was towards the sycotic miasm, with the colitis and urinary involvement.

Sepia has a strong miasmatic connection to sycosis and is a major remedy for female reproductive and urinary problems, but the impression given at the consultation was more of Natrum Muriaticum. It was accordingly prescribed, one dose of a 30c night and morning for three days. This produced some improvement in the energy levels, which were maintained, together with the appearance of more definite symptoms of cystitis accompanied by mucoid sediment and occasional small amounts of frank blood in the urine. Some nocturnal incontinence also appeared. However, both the urine blood and protein readings on the urine test had decreased (+). The Natrum Muriaticum was repeated at 30c for two days with the result that energy levels improving further, until there were now short spells when she felt 'almost normal'. The bowels and bladder were unchanged, although she could not be induced to stop taking the herbs. There was now also a tense and full feeling around the lower abdomen, not relieved by passing either motion or urine. A further blood test showed further improvement in the anaemia. A single dose of Natrum Muriaticum 200c was given but there was no further clinical change.

It was then revealed that in addition to feeling frustrated by her condition the lady also felt trapped by life generally. She regarded her job as the most important aspect of her life, but resented the fact that she was already reaching the top of her career structure.

Sepia 200c night and morning for three days was then given on the basis of this new insight into the mental state, and she was finally persuaded to stop taking the herbs. After one week there had been a further marked increase in energy, but the night time urinary frequency had changed to frank incontinence with complete lack of bladder sensation. Control was present during the day provided the bladder did not become too full. The urine, however, appeared normal. Her sleep was now being disturbed by a generalised skin irritation that commenced on undressing and continued in bed. The tenseness in the lower abdomen eased somewhat and the motions became very watery, although their passage was without any marked pain.

Causticum 30c was administered, night and morning for three days, essentially as a complementary remedy to Sepia, having strong indications for weakness of the bladder. This gave a 35% (patient's assessment) improvement in the incontinence, with some feeling of the need to urinate returning. Repetition of the remedy dose after two weeks resolved the incontinence. The sediment in the urine began reappearing on alternate days and then cleared over the following three weeks. The energy levels continued to improve until the patient considered that any tiredness was due to genuine work rather than illness. The night-time skin irritation became worse and the bowels were still consistently loose.

Because of the skin situation and symptoms, after one month three doses of Sulphur 30c were administered over twenty-four hours (consistent with the prescribing sequence of Sepia followed by Sulphur). This produced forty-eight hours of acute diarrhoea with great urgency, but no blood or mucus. After this the motions returned to complete normality in about ten days. The itching of the skin disappeared over approximately the same period. No further treatment was necessary.

Discussion

Although there were signs of all three miasms in this case, the pattern was predominantly sycotic with some psoric elements, such as the tiredness. The initial nephritis may well have been psoric, but the presenting picture of the irritable bowel followed by the urinary involvement was definitely sycotic. The effect of the herbal treatments on this progression is significant, as just because a treatment uses natural substances does not necessarily mean that its action is natural, and suppression can occur as a result of their use. The structure of the case pointed towards the choice of a predominantly sycotic/psoric remedy, and Natrum Muriaticum fitted both the pattern, the family history and the initial presenting picture. The effect was to concentrate the sycotic picture slightly, which, together with new information regarding the patient's mental state, led to the prescription of Sepia. That moved the balance once more, and the consequent change of emphasis in the case to psoric/sycotic was addressed by the Causticum. The picture became one of an increased psoric influence, which was then rounded off by Sulphur.

Chapter 9

Syphilis

Basic Concepts

In *Chronic Diseases* Hahnemann describes syphilis as 'the miasm of the venereal disease proper', and he appears to link the miasm to the known clinical disease more closely than is the case with the other two miasms. This is a case of Hahnemann being constrained by the clinical experience and terminology of his time. An unfortunate consequence of this perceived association is that many writers have overstressed the importance of what he described later in the same chapter of *Chronic Diseases* as 'impure coition' in the clinical development of the miasm (see Chapter 1). As with sycosis, although such a route of infection is undoubtedly significant, potentially it detracts from a true understanding of the nature of the miasm. In fact, Hahnemann was primarily concerned with the proper treatment of the venereal disease in order to avoid the establishment of the miasm as a clinical entity. He regarded primary syphilis as an easily curable disease, given correct systemic treatment rather than the erroneous concentration on the local symptoms so common in his day.

The ill effects of such treatment were well documented by his contemporaries and supported his contention that the serious consequences arose as a result of suppressive treatment, which resulted in both the establishment of the miasm in its own right and its combination with psora and sycosis. It was these latter combinations that produced the most intractable of the problems. Syphilis, if allowed to flourish to its tertiary stage, is one of the most destructive of diseases, affecting the whole body. Equally, the miasm is the most actively destructive of the three basic forces. Its very name derives from the Greek word *siphilos,* meaning to cripple or maim.

It may be regarded as having similarities to the Oxygenoid constitution of Grauvogl's classification, where there is considered to be either an excess of oxygen within the system or an undue influence of external oxygen on the metabolism. This results in a stimulated and overactive metabolism, with consequent destruction. The analogy of the effects of oxygen on a fire gives an indication of the activity of the miasm.

One apparent paradox is that while its manifestation is linked to destruction, before that occurs there may be great strength and resolve. Many of the substances from which the major syphilitic remedies are derived are metals or other substances that exhibit great strength and worth, and have fixed and rigid structures. With the miasm it is as if there are no half measures, and once the defences have been breached there is a rapid decline into complete destruction.

Clinical Manifestations

Clinically its effects are seen in those conditions characterised by the disruption, perversion and degeneration of both tissues and function. Weakness of joints, ataxia and failure of healing due to degeneration of tissues are manifestations of this. In many ways it is nature's 'self-destruct button', turning in on itself and destroying the very structures and functions on which life depends. It encompasses those states described as 'dys', as in dysplasia and dystrophy. Ulceration, suppuration, unresponsive chronic infection and necrosis arise from the miasm.

The syphilitic type often has problems and issues surrounding their own identity, and a love of travel is often found (Lilley, 2005). This may, in part, be a reflection of a desire to 'find themselves'. There may also be a feeling of unending suffering, with no end to their troubles (Sherr, 2002). Mentally there is often dullness, obstinacy and introversion, with an anxiety and restlessness that is hidden. There can be a lack of alertness and imagination and a slowness to take on new ideas. Idiocy and mental retardation are seen, being the ultimate destruction of the mental powers. At the same time there can be great drive and vision in an individual, but things must be done in exactly the way that they decree, and if this is checked for any reason then there can be a rapid descent into depression and self-condemnation. Strong feelings of guilt, self-loathing and uncleanness arise easily, and the 'self-destruct' aspect comes into play here with a strong tendency towards suicide. However, unlike other types, syphilitic patients will often not talk about suicide – they will just do it. The self-destructive urge may also manifest as addiction to either drugs or alcohol. The type has a natural tendency to keep their problems to themselves and brood on them, and it is almost as if the depression and burden finally becomes so great that something violent must be done to break out of the cycle, even if that something is the destruction of the self!

Violence generally, with little thought for the consequences, is also a feature of the type. There is much distrust, jealousy and cruelty, with a marked indifference to the sufferings of others, based in a lack of confidence both in other people and in the world generally. There is a feeling that only when *they* are in control will things run smoothly, and that control must be exercised at all costs. This feeling may be allied to a genuine love of power. Compulsive behaviour of various types is often seen, possibly as a means of protecting the individual from the perceived hostile world. The self-centred nature will result in a failure to abide by the accepted rules and conventions of society, or to interpret them in a highly individual way to their own benefit. Ruthless dictators are essentially syphilitic, and in the animal world the excessively dominant pack or herd leader is exhibiting the same trait.

Great fear and anxiety about many things is prominent in the picture, but a recurring theme is concern about health. This manifests as a fear of infection and becoming ill, linked to a despair of recovery. When added to the tendency towards compulsive behaviour, this leads to such patterns as obsessive hand-washing and excessive fixations that certain things or foods will do them harm. Severe pain can result in great depression, which in all species can produce loss of appetite and a withdrawal into themselves, and in humans may trigger suicide. All illness will induce some degree of depression in the syphilitic patient.

There is a marked time modality to the syphilitic miasm, with conditions being worse from sunset to sunrise. The conditions are also worse for physiological discharges, such as perspiration, but better for pathological discharges, as when pus finds an outlet. Extremes of temperature are disliked but there is a preference for cold foods and drink. There is a tendency for cold to ameliorate most symptoms. Movement and warmth will aggravate most conditions, which are also generally worse near the sea.

Pains may be intense, but conversely severe lesions may be painless, especially on the skin. Conventionally this may be explained by the fact that the degree of destruction is so great that the nerve endings themselves have been destroyed. Indeed in most syphilitic cases there will be destruction of normal tissue. Severe bone pains are experienced, especially at night, and in the long bones.

The senses and their organs are particularly susceptible to the miasm. Many eye problems have a strong syphilitic component, often with a photophobia that is worse for artificial light. Ophthalmia and blepharitis are seen, aggravated by heat and relieved by cold applications. The middle ear is prone to abscesses and bony destruction, and much of the ulceration in otitis externa is syphilitic. Infected nasal polyps and ulcerative destruction of the nasal septum are accompanied by a foul thick discharge. The presence of the miasm should be considered in all cases showing persistent nasal discharges. The function of all the senses can be lost, but this is due to destruction of the tissues rather than the pure failure of function, which is psoric.

Painful ulceration of the mouth with salivation and swelling of the tongue is seen. The imprint of the teeth on the tongue is seen in humans, although it is not observed to the same extent in animals. There is perversion of taste, with putrid or metallic sensations being reported. The caries associated with dental neck lesions are syphilitic in nature, and many abnormal developments of the teeth are also a result of the miasm. These are not the slow dentition of psora that finally gives a normal mouth, but rather a disjointed development that gives an uneven and ugly mouth of teeth. Abdominal pains are burning and tearing and tend to be intense. There is a strong desire for spicy foods and alcohol. Syphilitic dogs seem especially fond of wine, which produces diarrhoea. In humans there may be a dislike of meat (this is a physical aversion rather than a moral inclination towards vegetarianism), and the occasional carnivore is seen that dislikes meat. The diarrhoea of syphilis is foul-smelling and may contain undigested food, blood or pus.

The whole of the respiratory system can be affected, with soreness and ulceration. There is difficulty in swallowing with ulceration of the pharynx and tonsils. Destruction of lung tissue causes dyspnoea. The cough is harsh, producing little discharge.

Developmental abnormalities of the heart are seen, and valvular conditions caused by degeneration.

Physiological genital discharges are copious, with an unpleasant smell. Menses are often accompanied by bone pains as well as more local discomfort.

Many skin lesions occur near the joints, where there is much movement of the tissues. Fissures and ulceration, both painful and painless, are features. Eczema is characterised by thick, sticky, offensive pus. In syphilitic cases there is a tendency to ulcer formation, and the development of external ulceration is usually associated with a general improvement in the patient.

The course of syphilis as a disease results in the formation of an external chancre, and it is the suppression of this that results in the rapid development of the condition to the secondary and tertiary stages. The destruction that is a feature of the tertiary stage of the disease is mirrored in the miasm. Swelling and ulceration of glandular tissue is often seen. There is often very little pruritis associated with the skin lesions, although pus and blood may be present. Thick crusts are commonly seen in syphilitic skin lesions, as are discolourations of the skin. These are not the increases of pigmentation seen in sycotic states, but rather often circular areas of a red/brown colour. There is a loss of normal pigmentation.

The discharges of syphilis are acrid and almost invariably offensive in nature.

The miasm is involved in developmental faults of all kinds, but particularly those affecting the skeleton. There is to some degree an affinity with the reproductive system, and although this is not as great as in the case of the sycotic miasm, it may nevertheless be a significant factor in some situations. Problems arising from congenital deformity of the hips, especially the left, are usually syphilitic in origin, whereas the development of Perthes' disease is regarded commonly as indicative of a syphilitic influence from both sides of the family. Similarly the miasm should be suspected in those animal litters that show a high proportion of congenital faults. The exact deformity may not be the same in every individual animal within the litter, but it is the total proportion that is significant. A single deformity in an otherwise normal litter may well be psoric in origin.

Suppression of the syphilitic miasm drives the disease process primarily into the brain, causing depression, and into the bones. The meninges, liver and genital organs are also affected, as are the eyes and aorta to some degree.

The Syphilitic Miasm and the Immune System

Destruction in the broadest sense of the term is an integral part of the normal physiological processes of the body. Even the breaking down of complex chemicals in the normal reaction chains connected with the metabolism of hormones, enzymes, amino acids and so on can be viewed as a form of destruction. However, in all these situations it is a controlled and balanced process, resulting in some benefit to the body. The term 'constructive destruction' could well be applied here.

Such reactions also occur within the immune system, but in addition there are the frank destructive activities associated with the defences of the body against outside challenge, as opposed to the maintenance of homeostasis. Phagocytosis is one such activity, antigen neutralisation is another. But even in these situations the destructive property is controlled and directed for the good of the whole, within the context of the unfolding of the full dynamic of the disease process. If the natural order of the disease response is interfered with by inappropriate medicinal procedures, then the effect can be to accentuate the influence of the destructive processes.

As with the relationship between sycosis and the reproductive system, because the requirement of destruction and removal of foreign agents and antigens is so vital to the proper functioning of the immune system, that function will be maintained wherever possible. It may also lead to the system turning in on itself if the normal process of response to challenge is either blocked or circumvented. This will encourage the creation and activity of the syphilitic miasm within the immune system. The scope of immune function, involving as it does the whole body, means that the clinical results of this may be seen on either a local or general level. Autoimmune disease is primarily a syphilitic phenomenon. From the miasmatic point of view, such a mechanism may be involved in the creation of autoimmune disease following repeated vaccination, although it must not be thought that this is the only means whereby the situation can arise.

The appearance of a frank syphilitic influence implies the presence of psora manifesting as a lack of control and direction. Control and orchestration of function is, of course, inherent in the normal maintenance of homeostasis. It is inevitable that this aspect of the activity of the immune system will also be affected when the body is coping with an acute challenge. Thus it is not surprising that, when the normal balance of the immune system collapses, it is both the syphilitic and psoric miasms that are manifest. In *Chronic Diseases* Hahnemann stressed what he described as the 'awakening' of psora as a result of the incorrect treatment of primary syphilis, and also drew attention to the intractability of the resulting combination, stating that 'when complicated with developed psora, it is impossible to cure the venereal disease alone.'

Syphilis in Combination

It is in combination with the other miasms that the effects of syphilis are seen at their worst. Hahnemann – also in *Chronic Diseases* – identified the combination of psora and syphilis, which he described as 'a monster of a double disease', and stressed the difficulties of curing such a condition. Known as either *pseudo-syphilis* or *masked syphilis,* the outline of its treatment forms the basis of all treatment of mixtures of miasms, and has been discussed in Chapter 4. However, it is the combination of psora and syphilis, with some sycosis in the more permanent form that is now recognised as the Tubercular miasm, which can prove even more difficult to treat. The other situation in which syphilis in combination is seen as a potent clinical force is in cancer. The miasmatic make-up of neoplasia has also been discussed in Chapter 4, but in general terms the more malignant the pathology the greater the syphilitic influence will be.

Antisyphilitic Remedies

Syphilinum is the nosode of the syphilitic miasm, being derived from the discharge of a syphilitic chancre. It is also known as Lueticum, from the Latin word *lues,* originally meaning a plague or pestilence; it later became specifically linked to the disease of syphilis. Many of the metals are predominantly syphilitic in nature, with Aurum, Mercury and many of their salts being of major importance. Phytolacca, often described as the 'vegetable mercury', should always be remembered in the syphilitic context, and Stillingia Sylvatica is another plant remedy with a major syphilitic component. Fluorine represents a strong syphilitic tendency and its salts are well represented in the syphilitic group, while Fluoric Acid itself is a major syphilitic remedy. Gettysburg Water, in contrast to many of the other spa water remedies, has strong syphilitic tendencies especially for destructive conditions manifesting around the hips and lower spine (Saxton, 2004). In addition, Carcinosin, Cinnabaris, Hepar Sulphuris, Kali Bichromicum, Kali Sulphuricum, Kali Iodatum, Nitric Acid, Phosphorus, Silica, Stellaria Media, Thallium and Tuberculinum all have a significant syphilitic component. The violent destructive character of gunpowder is reflected in a strong syphilitic aspect to it as a remedy, whilst one of its constituents, Kali Nitricum, also shows syphilitic tendencies. (The explosive nature of gunpowder connects more to a sycotic signature, and in its material form was used by troops during the first world war as a self-help treatment for gonorrhoea.) Lachesis, although not in the first rank of antisyphilitic remedies, does have some significant effect in this direction.

CASE 11: *Pulmonary carcinoma*

A male Doberman was referred after a diagnosis by radiography and biopsy of pulmonary carcinoma. His exact age was unknown as he was originally a stray, but the estimate was around eleven years. He had been in his present home for eight years. When originally found he had been in very poor condition, with evidence of a badly healed fracture of the tenth rib on the left side. He had been nursed back to good health and there had been no subsequent major health problems up to eighteen months previously, when two lipomata were removed from the left flank at the owner's request. They had not been causing any clinical problems and were classed as lipomata on clinical examination, with no histopathology being performed. Six months later a dry cough developed, without any systemic illness. It was treated by the referring veterinary surgeon with a course of potentiated sulphonamide and appeared to resolve without any further problem. Some six weeks prior to the consultation the cough had returned and the sulphonamide was again given, this time with no effect. Although the dog was still eating well and was lively, the cough had steadily worsened. It was at this stage that investigations were undertaken and the diagnosis of carcinoma made. A very poor prognosis had been given, due to the extent of the lesion and the nature of the condition, and the only treatment option offered was palliative (involving steroids), until such time as the situation became untenable from the welfare point of view. His life expectancy had been quoted in weeks.

On clinical examination he appeared reasonably alert and interested in his surroundings, but the owners said that he was somewhat subdued and not his usual self. There was no marked respiratory embarrassment but the cough was < movement. It was also < from 10 p.m. but eased between 5–6 a.m. Auscultation revealed a large dull area in the left lung, and the trachea sounded harsh and dry. The right lung sounded normal. (The radiographs were unavailable.) A urine sample showed a ++ (on a scale of 1–4) reaction to protein on dipstick and a trace of blood. Apparently when he had returned home after the biopsy was taken there had been frank blood in the urine. This had been put down to cystitis, no treatment had been given, and it had resolved in a few days.

He was described as being very loyal to, and protective of, his owners. He liked people and got on well with the other dog in the house. He liked to be petted and was not aggressive, but showed some jealousy for the owners' attention. He would not play with balls or other toys, nor with the other dog. He disliked being on his own but was not destructive if left without company. He had a great fear of thunder and fireworks. He had always been restless at night and would wake the owners up, for no apparent reason, by going round to each and licking them, but he did not bark. On these occasions he did not wish to be let out for toilet purposes, but seemed merely to want to check that they were all there. After waking everyone up he wanted to be wrapped up in his bed again, when he would settle. These activities only occurred during the hours of darkness, irrespective of the season. One of the reasons that he was considered to be subdued was that this nocturnal behaviour had ceased and he was sleeping through the night. He loved heat in all forms. Both appetite and thirst had always been excessive and he would eat anything. Left to himself he would drink water to the point of making himself sick.

The strong laterality of the case, together with the thirst, love of heat, blood in urine, behaviour in the dark and love of company led to a prescription of Phosphorus, and this was administered at 30c night and morning for five days. Three weeks later he was more alert, and in the words of the owners 'was once more his usual self'. He had again started to wake all the family in the night (to their great delight!). The cough was unchanged, as were the lungs on auscultation. On testing there was no blood in the urine and the protein had reduced to +. Phosphorus 200c was then administered night and morning for two days. This produced a temporary improvement of the cough, which then regressed to its previous intensity and modality, and he once more stopped waking in the night.

Syphilinum 200c was then given daily for three days, as it was felt that a deeper-acting miasmatic remedy was needed, and the only clear modality was < night. This resulted in him becoming, as the owners described, 'the best he has been since he became ill'. The cough improved again, and virtually disappeared for a short time, but then recurred. Phosphorus 200c was repeated for three doses in twenty-four hours, with no further improvement, although the general situation was maintained, and the dog was otherwise his normal self. Bacillinum 30c one dose weekly for four weeks was then given as, in the author's experience, this is a particularly effective preparation of Tuberculinum where there is lung pathology. This controlled the cough but it returned immediately at the end of the course. Thereafter a weekly dose of Bacillinum maintained the situation for fourteen months before he collapsed and died. No post-mortem was carried out, and so the exact cause of death was not ascertained. However, given the life expectancy of a Doberman at twelve to thirteen years, the provision of quality life for the equivalent, in human terms, for three to four years may be considered a success, especially in view of the fact that the prognosis had been of only a few weeks to live at the outset of treatment.

Discussion

The approach to this case would probably have been very different in the human field.

The clear result from the biopsy was an instance where modern diagnostic techniques can be of help in a miasmatic interpretation of a case. A carcinoma implies a syphilitic/sycotic/psoric hierarchy in the case, and hence the indication for a strongly antisyphilitic remedy at the start. The overall clinical features at the initial presentation led to the selection of Phosphorus. The limited success of this led to the use of the miasmatic nosode related to syphilis, in an attempt to control the obviously overwhelming syphilitic factor in the case. Although the Bacillinum was used, essentially as a remedy directed at the specific respiratory symptoms, the fact that no other remedy was subsequently required raises the interesting possibility of what would have been the effect of using Tuberculinum initially. However, the high degree of syphilitic activity in the tubercular miasm means that there may have been a miasmatic overlap in this case. Indeed, some authorities class Phosphorus as a major antitubercular remedy (Banerjea, 1993). This was undoubtedly a case of a mixed miasm, and that, linked to the advanced degree of pathology present at the start of the homeopathic treatment, meant that palliation was all that could be achieved. The history of the removal of the 'lipomas' prior to the development of a more major condition raises the possibility that, miasmatically, they may not have been the benign entities that was assumed, and that their removal resulted in a suppression of the whole disease process. The procedure must be regarded as possibly having been suppressive.

Another treatment approach would have been the longer-term use of other miasmatic nosodes such as Carcinosin or Scirrhinum. However, the regime that was employed was providing adequate control, so a change would possibly have been counterproductive. Similarly, the repetition of Syphilinum was considered and rejected on the basis that the clinical situation was stable.

CASE 12: *An obstinate degeneration*

A fifty-two-year-old veterinary surgeon, the senior partner in the practice, sought help because of a persistent and intractable infection in the roots of the molar teeth on both sides of his upper jaw. He had had much dental work over the previous years, involving both extensive fillings and some extractions. The condition was essentially painless, but he did complain of intermittent tenderness around the mouth generally. The infection had been diagnosed by X-ray during ongoing dental procedures. Several courses of antibacterial agents had been given, including amoxycillin and metronidazole, all to no effect. He had been referred to a dental hospital for the current problem and their suggested solution had been extensive extractions. He was unwilling to follow this route and his dentist agreed, considering that bridge work would be feasible as an alternative if the infection could be cleared first.

The other ongoing problem was sinusitis, from which he had suffered for many years. This involved both sides of his face, with a somewhat greater intensity on the right, as opposed to the left, side. Virtually any exposure to severe weather conditions would bring on an attack, with copious yellow-green discharge from the nostrils, usually accompanied, as the condition progressed, by pus and blood. The blood came away intermittently in dark clots with a strong smell, rather than as epistaxis. There was never any suggestion of the chest being involved in any way, no matter how severe the sinusitis. There were occasional episodes of bleeding from the gums but no persistent gingivitis. The facial areas over the sinuses were sensitive to touch during the attacks, which also produced great depression in the patient, who was normally of an extremely forceful and exuberant nature. This depression appeared to be more than just the effect of pain, as a previous health scare some two years previously, involving the painless enlargements of some superficial lymph nodes, had produced exactly the same psychological effect. This, fortunately, had come to nothing of apparently lasting consequence and had been resolved with antibiotics, after which his usual good humour had been restored.

Antibiotics, in fact, had featured largely in the medical history of the case, as every attack of sinusitis had been treated with them, and a whole range had been used over the years. Other than that there had been two problems. One was a tendency to headaches, which could affect either or both sides, and which were aggravated during, but not confined to, the attacks of sinusitis. The other was occasional episodes of what were described as 'sciatica' involving the left leg, and for which no clear aetiology or modality could be established. Analgesics and anti-inflammatories had been used as had seemed appropriate. His only previous exposure to homeopathy had been the successful use of Mezereum following a mercury amalgam filling that caused great pain, prescribed because of the pains in the teeth at the time and the known effect of the remedy in antidoting the ill effects of Mercury.

Gunpowder 30c night and morning for five days was prescribed, based on the presence of a persistent infection and the right-sided predominance of the sinusitis. Coccal Co. was also considered, as being a remedy in its own right for persistent low-grade sepsis, but was rejected as it was felt that the case was essentially syphilitic rather than tubercular. Coccal Co. reflects the tubercular miasm, as the fact that its only associated remedy is Tuberculinum indicates (Paterson, 1949). The Gunpowder was stopped after forty-eight hours because of an acute flare-up of the sinusitis, accompanied by a feeling of tightness in the chest that had not been present before. This latter resolved in twenty-four hours without treatment. The patient was persuaded not to resort immediately to antibiotics and the sinusitis settled over three to four days.

It was not thought advisable to repeat the Gunpowder because of the appearance of the new symptom – the sensation of tightness in the chest – following its previous administration, and so Mezereum 30c night and morning was given for five days, on the basis of the mental reactions to the problems, the presence of infection in the tooth roots and the proven success of the remedy previously. Although there were no obvious clinical effects, further X-rays of the teeth three weeks later showed an improvement in the situation. Mezereum 30c once daily for one week was then administered. The long-term effects of the treatment were that the infection cleared, as demonstrated by further X-rays, and the required dental work was successfully carried out without the need for extractions; the sinusitis attacks continued but without the bleeding and frank pus, and without causing the same depression. Unfortunately, in spite of his experiences, the patient remained firmly committed to his allopathic convictions and would not pursue the further possibilities offered! However, the improvement in his mouth and head generally was maintained for at least some two years, until contact was lost with him.

Discussion

Although there is undoubtedly some sycosis present, the theme of syphilis runs overwhelmingly through this case, with the general dental weakness and the suppressed infections associated with it. The mental reaction to illness generally is also syphilitic, with the sudden collapse, albeit temporary, of a strong character. The sinusitis undoubtedly had a sycotic component, as shown by the copious nasal discharge associated with the attacks, but the blood and pus present in the condition were indicative of a syphilitic influence. The overall attitude of the patient, with his continuing commitment to the orthodox wisdom and consequent unwillingness to envisage a new approach, had dictated the essentially local prescribing for the presenting problem. Both Gunpowder and Mezereum are leading syphilitic remedies with sycotic components, and the successful use of the latter on a previous occasion where there had been an aetiology involving a material syphilitic substance in the form of a mercury-based amalgam, is an interesting aspect of the case. The suppressive effect of the numerous courses of antibiotics will inevitably have had an influence on the development of this condition.

CASE 13: *A destructive injury*

A twelve-year-old Arab cross mare lived on a farm with one other horse, a gelding (neutered male), both being used for purely recreational riding by the family. She was of average build and was 15.1 hands at the withers (1 hand = 4 inches, therefore 5' 1"). She was friendly to people and other horses, a willing worker, but somewhat nervous of unknown things when they were first encountered, and she could panic even at a plastic bag blowing in the wind. She was not keen on wind, rain, or extreme heat but was otherwise indifferent to weather. Her appetite was basically good, thirst unremarkable, and bowel action was normal. Oestrus was normal, and as far as was known she had had two foals before coming to her present home some two years previously. She had been wormed and vaccinated regularly.

Some six months prior to the consultation she had been found in the field with a wound on the right hand side of the face, just above and medial to the eye. There was no known cause and it was presumed that she had panicked at something and as a result had run headlong into one of the trees in the field. She was fully conscious and investigation revealed a depressed and fragmented fracture of the frontal bone with extensive bruising of the area. The eye was involved in the general soft tissue reaction but there was no permanent tissue damage to the area. Arnica had been given immediately the situation had been discovered and appreciated by the owner. Subsequently surgery, accompanied by anti-inflammatory drugs and antibiotics was used to treat the injury and repair, as far as possible, the skeletal integrity. The recovery from the general anaesthetic and the wound healing were uneventful, leaving a depressed area visible on the skull that gave no clinical problems. Arnica had been administered by the owner both pre- and post-operatively. There had been no behavioural changes following the incident, but the horse had never fully regained the general physical condition she had before it, and her appetite had remained only adequate.

Some three months after the accident a unilateral discharge appeared from the right nostril. This was green in colour, thick, and generally moderate in quantity. Although initially intermittent, it increased in frequency until it became present at all times, with no observed modality. Every four to five days there would be bouts of sneezing, resulting in the appearance of larger clots of the discharge mixed with blood, and what the owner described as 'pieces of flesh'. It was presumed that these were pieces of nasal mucosa. Once this had come away, the sneezing ceased until the next clot built up and was discharged in a similar manner. The frequency of these attacks was not increasing. Three courses of antibiotics had no long-term beneficial effect on the discharge, the only effect being a slight temporary easing after the first course.

Although still eating, and with no difficulty, there had been further reduction of the appetite, and the horse had began to lose both weight and condition steadily, with her coat becoming dull, containing much dandruff and with the hair falling out. Faecal examination found no worms, the teeth were normal, and a blood sample revealed no abnormality. There was no diarrhoea. Anabolic steroids failed to halt the deterioration in the general condition. At the same time an apparently bony lump, about the size of an egg, developed immediately above the site of the injury. Throughout all this the patient remained reasonably responsive, but continued to eat poorly and was not as bright as she had been before the incident.

On examination there was no pain around the head, and no enlargement of the cervical lymph glands. The lump was hard, appeared attached to the underlying bone, and was painless on palpation. There was a low-grade conjunctivitis in the right eye, with a slight pale green discharge. Auscultation of the trachea and lungs showed them to be normal.

Mercurius Solubilis 30c was prescribed night and morning for five days on the basis of the nature of the nasal discharge. Two weeks later that discharge had, overall, become less, was more intermittent, and there had been no further episodes of sneezing. The horse was more alert and eating a bit better, but still losing condition. Merc. Solubilis 200c was administered night and morning for three days. After this the discharge ceased completely and the appetite improved back to the level that it had been at prior to the onset of the discharge. Although the loss of condition ceased, it only improved slightly and the increased appetite did not produce any significant weight gain. Gaertner Bach 200c night and morning for five days was given, both on the indication of the failure to thrive in spite of the other improvements, and because of its association with the remedy (Mercury) which had produced those improvements that there had been. After three weeks there was a noticeable improvement in the general condition, which continued for a further two weeks but then stopped. However, there was no regression and such improvement as there had been was maintained. Gaertner Bach 200c was repeated night and morning for two days and the improvement resumed. The discharge had not returned but the lump on the face was unchanged. Hecla Lava 30c night and morning was prescribed because of the presence of an exostosis on the face, in spite of the fact that there was no pain (which symptom the author considers to be unreliable in relation to Hecla Lava). A ten-day course reduced the size of the facial lump by about one-third. Subsequent courses as necessary removed it completely in six weeks, by which time complete normality had been restored.

Discussion

The development of an apparently bony lump and the accompanying discharge might initially have been thought to make the case sycotic, due to the new tissue growth and the evidence of increased mucosal discharges. However, the picture of the initial injury and the violent nature of the presumed cause pointed to a destructive theme running through the case. As indicated in Chapter 3, the author's view is that the intrinsic character of any individual challenge reflects a balance of the basic forces of nature, which are expressed in the body as production, removal and control. As such, the resonance induced in the body by a particular challenge will mirror that individual balance of forces, and hence influence the nature of the body's response. This was reflected here in the syphilitic nature of the symptoms, namely the nasal bleeding with loss of tissue, which indicated a degree of ulceration of the nasal mucosa. The loss of condition immediately following the injury and its treatment was unremarkable, but it was more the failure to thrive once that period was over, and especially once the other improvements had begun, that was miasmatically significant. The Kali salts were considered, particularly Kali Bichromicum and Kali Iodatum, due to the nature of the nasal discharges, but the total pictures did not fit as well, and the overview of the case indicated the choice of an even stronger antisyphilitic remedy. Hence Mercury was prescribed. Gaertner Bach has the keynote of 'malnutrition', especially when the cause is associated with the bowels (Paterson, 1949), as well as being linked to both Mercury and the syphilitic miasm. Hecla Lava as a more local prescription was chosen rather that Silica, primarily on the basis of the bony enlargement being on the face. Silica was considered, due to it being a leading associated remedy of Gaertner Bach, and its remedy picture being described as forming part of that of Gaertner Bach. However, Hecla Lava, as indicated above, appeared to be the more appropriate remedy, which, as events proved, matched the miasmatic influence in the case at that time. Although Hecla Lava has a syphilitic aspect to it, it also has a significant sycotic element that could be used to address the more local pathology.

Chapter 10

The Miasmatic Nosodes

There are many nosodes in the homeopathic materia medica, but not all can be classed as miasmatic nosodes. Many of them, such as Morbillinum obtained from measles and Distemperinum from canine distemper, are derived from cases of acute infections. Anthracinum, the first nosode to be produced, was created from the spleen of a bovine case of anthrax which Hahnemann classified as belonging to the group of acute miasms. Lyssin (Hydrophobinum) produced using the saliva of a rabid dog as the source material was similarly called a 'half-acute' miasm. (See Chapter 3 for a discussion of the difference between acute and chronic miasms.)

In contrast, the so-called miasmatic nosodes are all derived from material produced by the body in situations where the clinical disease is one of those identified with the main miasms, and hence where the respective miasmatic pattern is strongly represented. Many of the symptoms will be found replicated in individual remedies associated with the particular miasms, as in the case of Sulphur and Psorinum, or Thuja and Medorrhinum. The concept of the miasmatic nosode representing the 'centre-point' of the miasm (Sankaran, 1994) is helpful in understanding why this is so. It is as if the miasm (represented in the nosode) produces the broad canvas, and the remedies account for the detail and variations around the central theme. It is because of this relationship that the miasmatic nosodes have uses over and above those of other remedies. Individual symptoms will be found in the remedy pictures that correspond to the themes of miasms other than the dominant one represented in the remedy. It must be remembered that what are being described here are remedies, not miasms, and this apparent paradox is an example of one aspect of the model presented in this book, namely that *in every situation and remedy, all three basic forces are always present to some degree.*

In general terms nosodes are used in either a homeopathic or an isopathic way. As in other situations involving a homeopathic prescription, the guiding principle is the presenting syndrome. Thus Distemperinum is used in cases of idiopathic epilepsy, not because this condition is caused by the distemper virus but because there are convulsions in the remedy picture of that nosode. Isopathic use involves the principle of 'same cures same' rather than the 'like (similar) cures like (similar)' of true homeopathy. Hahnemann, in the footnote to Paragraph 56 of the *Organon* cautions against this approach in acute situations. However, the use of nosodes in the case of chronic illness is not isopathy as defined, as it is not attempting to cure the named disease with which it is associated. It is a way of addressing the totality of the disease picture.

Miasmatic nosodes can be used in various ways. Firstly it must be remembered that they are remedies in their own right, with their own symptom pictures, and that they can always be prescribed on that presenting picture. Another important use is as intercurrent remedies based on the miasmatic interpretation of a case. Used in this way they will often unblock a case and allow other indicated remedies to complete their action. Cases will also be seen where cure has progressed to the final stages in accordance with Hering's Law, but the symptoms remain stuck at the body's extremities in spite of further well-selected remedies. An appropriate miasmatic nosode may well resolve these cases. The nosodes may also be used with advantage when a symptom picture presents that contains many contradictory elements. They are deep-acting remedies, often addressing the inherited miasmatic situation whilst other remedies act on the acquired aspects of the case. In the treatment of conditions involving mixed miasms, they can be invaluable as a means of counteracting the unified but essentially unbalanced action of the fixed functional forces that are active in these situations (see Chapter 4).

There may be an understandable reluctance to start a case with a miasmatic nosode in the absence of a clear symptom picture pointing to it as a remedy in its own right, but too much caution can be exercised in these situations. If there is a good match, then the nosode is being used as a remedy in its own right. If no clear remedy picture presents but there is a definite miasmatic pattern, then the appropriate nosode can indeed be used as the first prescription, as there will be a definite connection to the underlying dynamic of the disease. Care should be exercised over the choice of potency, with a moderate level being employed, but this is only following the general prescribing rule where there are no very individually specific symptoms. Mention has been made in Chapter 6 of the possible use of miasmatic nosodes in a preventive role.

Since, like all true nosodes, those discussed below originate from sources associated with an active disease process, they all contain that all-important component, the energy imprint of the body's reaction to the challenge to which it has been exposed (Hallamaa et al, 2001). The use of autogenous nosodes (autopathy) represents one means of utilising that imprint in a specific way, with the nosode and a remedy often being used together. This is in contrast to remedies prepared from pure cultures of infective agents, such as Streptococcinum and Staphylococcinum, or from vaccines as in the case of the canine and feline preparations, which often are referred to (incorrectly) as nosodes. The term pathode should be applied to these preparations. Since consideration of the miasms is essentially a consideration of the *functional* aspects of disease, this dimension of the body's response which is present in the true nosodes adds significantly to the usefulness of these agents.

Psorinum

As the name implies, this is associated with the psoric miasm, the source material being the discharge from a vesicle in a case of scabies. As has been seen in Chapter 4, the essence of psora is deficiency and upset of function, and the remedy reflects these characteristics throughout its picture. The patient may present with a whole range of symptoms but with very little pathology. The picture shows the mental anxiety of the miasm, with delusions, dreams and fears of illness, failure – especially in business – and poverty. This is equated in the animal world with the excessive and unnecessary hoarding of food, such as the dog that is adequately and regularly fed still burying bones and other portions of its food. Depression, guilt and feelings of being abandoned may be so great as to engender thoughts of suicide. Such thoughts, however, are unlikely to be acted on. Linked to the depression there is often an unwillingness to act, even when action would be in the sufferer's own best interests. This is also seen on the physical level as a general lack of reactivity and failure to regain vitality following illness, with a despair of recovery. It also leads to the failure of other well-selected remedies to act, and this may be overcome by the intercurrent use of the nosode. The failure of remedies selected on the aetiological basis of 'never well since' should always lead to consideration of the psoric nosode. One unusual feature is that the patient will often feel particularly well just prior to illness manifesting, and may display a ravenous appetite at that time.

There is a general weakness, and effort of any kind, either mental or physical, tends to produce an aggravation. Copious perspiration may occur on the slightest exertion, or even at rest. There is great sensitivity to external stimuli, and it is a major remedy in the treatment of allergies. As might be expected, there is extreme chilliness in the picture, with a corresponding great desire for heat. This results in the seeking out and monopolising of any source of heat, and also in a desire to be covered up. Many animals are unable to lie out in the sun, but this may be due as much to being outside, which can aggravate conditions, rather than dislike of the sun. Animals will burrow under bedding, burying their heads as well as their bodies. People will never be without a hat of some type, and there is a great sensitivity to draughts. A strong feature is a general worsening by cold and a tendency to catch colds, although paradoxically, in spite of the great need for warmth, many conditions are made worse by heat. Generally, as might be expected, the type is worse in the winter and better in the summer. Changes in the weather can be detrimental. All pathological discharges are offensive and tend towards a putrid odour.

Headaches are accompanied by feelings of fullness in the skull, and are often linked to upsets in vision.

The eyes show redness of both the sclera and the tissues surrounding the eye, with chronic inflammation, soreness and acrid discharges. There is photophobia for both natural and artificial light.

The mouth shows ulceration of the gums and tongue and swelling of the throat. The tongue and soft palate in humans are coated in white mucus, although this is often not seen in animals to the same degree. There is a putrid taste in the mouth. Appetite is generally very good but may not return after acute illness. There is a desire to eat in the middle of the night, but in spite of eating well the patient will remain thin. Thirst is generally good. In spite of what may be a ravenous appetite and a generally catholic taste, there is an aversion to pork. There is nausea and belching with the smell of rotten eggs. Cramping abdominal pains are relieved by passing offensive flatus. There may be constipation or dark-coloured, very strong-smelling diarrhoea which may contain mucus and some blood. Constipation may be difficult to overcome, and there may be difficulty in passing even a soft motion, although diarrhoea is passed without much straining.

Respiratory conditions tend to be recurring, especially in the winter. The cough is dry and triggered by tickling in the larynx. Conditions are characterised by shortness of breath and are < cold and open air. Heart murmurs are seen and there is a weak pulse. All respiratory and cardiac conditions are > lying down or being still.

Skin symptoms figure largely in the Psorinum picture, and its use should be considered at some stage in all longstanding skin conditions. There is usually intense irritation which causes the patient to become mentally depressed. The irritation is such that the patient will often scratch until they make the skin bleed. The skin may appear coarse and dry, or there can be crustiness and vesicles producing a thin yellow exudate. The lesions occur all over the body and tend to bleed easily. Alopecia will often be seen. The whole skin can have an unhealthy look about it, and although dryness is the overriding feature there may be some greasiness due to excessive secretions by the sebaceous glands. This overactivity of the glands can lead, in dogs and cats, to problems with the anal glands, which often become chronically infected. There is a tendency for wounds and skin lesions to become infected, and even when wounds stay clean they will only heal slowly.

Discharges from the ears are brown to red, offensive and watery. Otitis is accompanied by great irritation, with rawness of the skin both in and around the ears.

Another marked feature of the remedy is the strong offensive smell associated with all aspects of it. There can be an unpleasant, usually musty smell from the body even when the patient is healthy, and all attempts to remove this by bathing have only a very temporary effect, only a few hours in many cases. Eruptions around the nails and on the feet may make walking difficult and painful.

The bladder is weak, which leads to incontinence, especially at night, and the need to pass water frequently at all times. Sexual function in both sexes is often irregular and poor, and females are generally < pregnancy.

Psorinum is in the list of remedies associated with the bowel nosode Morgan Pure (see below). Where Bacillinum has proved of benefit in the acute aspects of a case, it is often Psorinum that will take the case forward by addressing the more chronic aspects of the condition. It is hence known as the chronic of Bacillinum.

Medorrhinum

Sycosis is represented by this nosode, which is prepared from the discharge of a patient suffering with gonorrhoea. Another more recent proving, involving meditation, has been carried out, resulting in the remedy Medorrhinum Americana (Evans, 1996). This is similar to the original remedy in many ways and is described as 'a remedy which encompasses but goes much deeper than the old', and is claimed to be of particular value in children. The following is from the standard proving and clinical experience.

Although symptoms can be marked, they often present on a narrow range representing a particular condition. The excesses associated with the miasm feature prominently in the remedy picture, and there can be extremes of behaviour and character, even within the same patient. As would be expected, there is a strong connection with the genital and urinary systems, and much pathology is seen there. The type is often sad and anxious, with mental confusion and delusions of failure, insanity and eternal damnation, which may tip over into aggression. Obsessive behaviour may be another response to the delusions. Everything seems unreal, as if the patients were outside themselves looking in; they anticipate events, and a degree of clairvoyance may be experienced. There is impatience and a great need to hurry, to the detriment of performing tasks well, which results in mental confusion and poor memory. There is derangement of the sense of time and it often seems to pass very slowly. There may be a feeling that someone is looking over their shoulder and staring at them. This delusion can be seen in animals, who will suddenly stop for no apparent reason and look round behind them, occasionally even snapping at the air.

The excesses of the miasm also show in the profuse nature of the discharges, which arise from the stimulation and irritation of any mucous surface. The discharges are thick, acrid, and irritant.

There is the general sycotic modality of < between sunrise and sunset, but there is an aggravation between 3–4 a.m. Medorrhinum is described as a hot remedy, meaning that the patient has an intrinsic internal warmth, and this can result in an aggravation of symptoms from heat. In the case of Medorrhinum there is also some aggravation from cold. The greatest adverse effect is from damp, although there are occasions when there is some amelioration. Another strong feature is amelioration at the seaside, and this includes both being near and in the sea. Thunderstorms produce general aggravation.

Joints are also involved in the excessive process, with much arthritis in the picture. The joints are swollen and tender to the touch, with sensations of burning in the extremities. Often the problems are confined to one joint only, with the knees (stifles) being particularly involved. Chronic spinal problems may well benefit from the nosode, as there is the same connection to symptoms affecting the back in the Medorrhinum picture as is seen in relation to the skin with Psorinum. As with the extremities, the back pain is burning. Longstanding cases involving joints will show exostoses. There is some amelioration by motion and this can show as restlessness with a constant changing of position, but prolonged movement often results in aggravation.

Pains of all types in all systems are found in the picture. Symptoms are generally better for lying on the abdomen. The classic 'knee-chest' or 'prayer' position is also seen, with the rear end being elevated while the head is kept on the ground. This position involves a degree of stretching and arching of the back, which also ameliorates the conditions.

Cramps and spasms occur in both the stomach and intestines, giving abdominal pains and colic. There is a large thirst and a dislike of cold food and drink. Diarrhoea is thin and contains mucus, and is accompanied by abdominal pain.

Much thick yellow mucus is produced in the throat and nose. There are suffocating feelings in the chest, with difficulty breathing. Some relief is obtained by sticking the tongue out, but this is not a reliable symptom in animals, especially in those species that do not sweat and hence rely more on panting for heat exchange.

Renal colic is seen. There is copious urination with straining involving both bladder and bowels when it is passed. Enlargement of the prostate in males is seen, together with discharge from the urethra, which may be thick yellow or thin and watery; both will stain material. Severe period pains are experienced in the female, with soreness of the mammary glands, which often feel cold to the touch at the time. Both sexual desire and function are high in both sexes, although the opposite is occasionally seen.

The skin exhibits a variety of benign pathologies, from the typical figwarts associated with the miasm to lipomata and cysts. There can be intense irritation with little sign of lesions. Changes in pigmentation occur, with an increase in those areas worse affected by pruritis. Healed lesions can leave either de-pigmented or brown coloured areas on the skin. Animals with musculoskeletal conditions often have feet with a strongly offensive smell as a concomitant symptom.

It is an associated remedy of the bowel nosode Morgan Pure. It is of particular use to complete the action of Lycopodium in males and Pulsatilla in females, especially if there are clear urinary symptoms in the disease picture.

Syphilinum (Lueticum)

The destruction and perversion associated with the syphilitic miasm is seen clearly in the remedy picture of the nosode. Violence is present, which will on occasion be directed outwards but is more often turned inwards against itself. There is thus an antisocial aspect, with bad temper tipping over into violent rages and a desire to kill. At the same time there may be an aversion to company through lack of confidence and depression, while feelings of worthlessness can lead to self-mutilation. Many fears are seen, which may be very general but tend to be specifically about health and death. There is constant worry both about becoming ill and recovering from illness. Behaviour patterns include the checking and rechecking of actions and situations, and there is a great attachment to superstitious practices.

As well as adhering to the generally accepted superstitions, such as not walking under ladders or touching wood, Syphilinum patients will invent their own rituals in which they find great comfort. This obsessive behaviour pattern, linked to the fear of disease and contamination, results in the characteristic feature of always washing the hands and a conviction that they are constantly dirty. On the mental level there is a desire to avoid involvement, and the constant washing of the hands can be interpreted by analogy as an attempt to shed responsibility. Another defence is to concentrate their energies on a narrow range of activities that they then feel they have mastered, and are therefore secure.

The self-destructive urge also finds expression in alcoholism and addiction to drugs, and the nosode is one of the major remedies for the treatment of these conditions.

The destructive theme is also seen in the physical symptoms of the nosode. There is extreme emaciation accompanied by a reduced or variable appetite. A major keynote is ulceration, which does not heal easily and may occur anywhere in the body. Recurring abscesses are a feature, and all discharges are putrid, with green pus.

Much saliva is produced in the mouth, with redness and ulceration of the mucosa. Swallowing anything may be difficult because of the degree of ulceration, which can affect all the tissues of the mouth. There is an aversion to meat, and the appetite is variable. There may be persistent vomiting due to ulceration of the alimentary tract while at the other end of the system there is an obstinate constipation. Flatulence is present due to dyspepsia, and there is painless diarrhoea, which is dark and foul-smelling.

In the eyes, chronic blepharitis, ophthalmia, iritis, keratitis and corneal ulceration are seen. The lids are red and swollen and there is severe photophobia. The lids may be stuck together in the morning.

Nasal discharges are thick, yellow and strong-smelling. Pressure on the throat triggers a harsh dry cough. Ulceration of the larynx and nasal mucosa is seen. Mucus accumulation in the chest produces moist râles.

There is intense pain in the ears with a watery, acrid and purulent discharge.

Pustular eruptions on the skin heal, leaving scars which are brownish in colour; while as fast as some heal others break out. The skin may have a blue tinge to it, while the irritation associated with the lesions may be less than would be expected.

The testicles are swollen and painful; there is sensitivity of all female genitalia with painful irregular periods producing thin, watery, acrid discharges.

Destructive pathology of the bones and teeth is seen. Ulceration of the nasal bones and tooth decay around the gums, both accompanied by offensive discharges, occurs. 'Dental neck lesions' in cats will often respond to Syphilinum (Viljoen, 1999). Destruction of long bones occurs while locomotor ataxia is seen. There are pains in the limbs and spine, with great stiffness, especially around the lumbar and sacral areas.

The strongest feature of the nosode is a marked aggravation of all symptoms at night, when pains and fears can become intense. There is consequently a fear of the night itself. Great weakness is seen in patients in the morning. In contrast to Medorrhinum, an aggravation at the seaside is usual. There is an aggravation from damp generally. It is essentially a chilly remedy, but is worse for either extreme of heat or cold. Local conditions are > applied heat.

Gaertner Bach is the associated bowel nosode. Syphilinum is the chronic of Mercurius and Nitric Acid.

Tuberculinum

This is one of the most widely indicated of the miasmatic nosodes in all species. Various forms have been prepared over the years by different authorities, using a range of tissues, or the isolated bacillus itself. Tuberculinum Bovinum, originating from the tubercular lung and lymph glands of a cow, and Tuberculinum Koch, based on a pure culture of the human bacillus, are the standard ones in common use. All other preparations conform to the same basic picture, with minor differences being claimed by their proponents. The view has been expressed (Gregory, 2003) that Tuberculinum Aviare (or Avis), from a tubercular chicken, has a more gentle action than other forms when used to treat skin conditions in animals. Bacillinum was produced using lung material from a human case of tuberculosis, and is widely considered to be particularly effective in longstanding and recurrent respiratory conditions.

The tubercular miasm was originally known as *pseudo-psora,* and is generally thought of as being a mix of psora and syphilis. However, the sycotic contribution is not insignificant and should not be forgotten. Tuberculosis as the clinical disease is a chronic, progressive and debilitating condition and these characteristics are mirrored in the nosode. Intermittent fevers, chronic respiratory conditions, recurrent infections, all with great weakening of the system, will often respond. When symptoms occur in the mid-line the tubercular influence should always be considered.

Restlessness and changeability are the keynotes of the remedy. Mentally this shows as a desire for new things and experiences. It is not necessarily a deep dissatisfaction with the status quo *per se*, but often rather a developing boredom and a 'wondering if the grass is greener' or 'change for the sake of change' mentality. A constant desire to travel, and refusal to be pinned down in any situation, are typical tubercular traits. Dogs that insist on escaping and roaming are often tubercular. On the other hand there may be an appearance of great stability in life, but within this solid framework the type finds its outlet by continuous changes of interests and hobbies. Tubercular people will thus often acquire a superficial knowledge of many things but with no ability to concentrate on any one thing in depth, while animals will often display an insatiable curiosity and desire to involve themselves with every object, person, or situation that comes their way.

The changeability also shows in the rapid alteration of moods, and swinging between a normally stable temperament and a violent outburst of temper, which may be triggered by the slightest thing. There is a general sensitivity to all impressions, including music. The expression of temper may not be purely verbal, but may feature malicious damage, especially in the young. Hyperactivity and a resentment of discipline are seen in both children and young animals. (Bacillinum has the symptom of initially defying discipline, and dogs will continue to grumble or growl even when it is enforced.) Fears do not feature prominently in the picture, although there is a vague fear that ‘something will happen’. The major fear in people is a fear of animals, particularly dogs. In the case of animals this is not reversed into a fear of people, but rather continues to manifest as a fear of other animal species.

Mental and physical symptoms may alternate, often rapidly. Within the physical dimension symptoms can also change swiftly, but usually within the same system. Symptoms are < closed room, cold and damp, draughts, noise and on waking; and > heat, open air and movement. These latter may in part be a reflection of the dislike of being confined or oppressed. Tuberculinum is a chilly remedy, but yet it will seek the open air. The type always feels cold during a fever and wants to be covered.

The appetite is often capricious, with constant changes of diet being demanded. Even when the appetite is good there is no weight gain, and in illness there is marked emaciation. Aphthae are seen in the mouth. Intractable diarrhoea occurs in the young. Diarrhoea may be sudden in onset and linked to vomiting and colic with burning and stinging pains, whilst the motion will be dark, offensive and forcibly expelled. The desire for smoked meats and alcohol reflects the need for stimulation, while milk is either loved or hated and may produce an allergic reaction. When it is craved it is usually preferred cold, and ice-cream may also be desired. There is a general desire for fats, sweets and salty tastes, and there may also be an aversion to meat. An individual may have a sensitivity to a particular food but at the same time will have a craving for that food.

The respiratory system is a major area of influence. The sense of not wanting to be confined in any situation for too long finds a parallel here with feelings of suffocation and shortness of breath, not only in an enclosed space, but even on occasion in the open. There is a desire for cool air and the wide open spaces. Respiration may be rapid even when there is no overt respiratory disease. Nasal discharges are yellow to green and contain mucus. There is inflammation of the throat, with a tickling feeling causing a dry cough. Tonsils are enlarged and the lymph nodes of the neck are indurated. There is a tendency to develop colds easily.

The eyelids are affected, with eczema on their margins. The ears show a persistent offensive discharge, with pains running from the ears to the pharynx. Otitis is accompanied by toothache.

There are wandering, aching pains in the joints and limbs and stiffness on first movement. Patients are < cold and damp and > heat and motion. On the mental level there is often a liking for, and a feeling of wellbeing when near, pine trees.

A sticky sediment is found in the urine, due to urates and mucus. Haematuria is accompanied by renal pain.

There are irregularities of the female sexual cycle, and the flow in all species is usually excessive and longlasting. The pains of the tubercular period increase when the flow starts.

The other area in which Tuberculinum is often called for is the skin. Allergic reactions fit the tubercular pattern of sudden and intense flaring of symptoms, and atopy is a major indication. Skin symptoms are < bathing. They are also < cold (undressing) but the pruritis is > heat. There is a dry skin with intense irritation and dandruff. Scratching moves the irritation to a new site. Eczema in the young is an indication. The use of Bacillinum in ringworm infections is a reflection of the sycotic element in the picture.

Carcinosin

The basic source material here is tissues from a cancerous human breast; in histopathological terms the lesion probably equates to an adenocarcinoma. In view of the role of suppression in the aetiology of cancer (see Chapter 8), it is not surprising that the remedy picture contains much that is associated with both control and the breaking free from control.

The remedy is often presented as one of contrasting extremes, between good and evil, order and chaos, high morality and base nature, and although this dichotomy exists to some degree in many remedies, it is particularly marked in the case of Carcinosin. Thus patients may be susceptible to both ends of the temperature range, although the tendency is to be more adversely affected by heat. The influence of the seaside is generally strong, and may either be to aggravate or ameliorate, although there is usually a sleeplessness associated with being near the sea. Liking for certain foods, such as salt and eggs, may change inexplicably to dislike (the desire for sweet things is usually more constant). Symptoms may change from side to side.

A temporary relief is obtained by the *release* of control, resulting in a marked enjoyment of thunderstorms and fireworks, a love of dancing and rhythmic movement, and a love of travel. Temporary *loss* of control, when it occurs, results in destructive outbursts and antisocial behaviour. Nevertheless, the picture that is usually seen is one of discipline and order, with fastidiousness and conscientiousness, which in part helps to hide a lack of confidence, sensitivity to criticism, and a degree of indecisiveness. There is usually a strong sense of duty. Mentally there can be the capacity for giving great sympathy and empathy, but there is tight control of emotions and actions, which may be self-generated or imposed from outside, as in the case of a highly-trained working animal of whom much is expected, or a child who is given too much responsibility too young.

Another aspect of this is that the animal or child will often only receive praise or attention when it has performed up to expectations, and the conditioning is thus established that love is dependent on performance. The element of control may be so strong that there is the delusion that the patient is under supernatural control (Squire, 1999). A marked love of animals is often seen in people. There is a general sensitivity with many fears and much anticipatory anxiety, which easily swing into guilt and depression.

On the surface the mental picture may resemble Pulsatilla. There is a similar desire to receive sympathy, but Carcinosin is not as soft and yielding, and has not the openness, of the true Pulsatilla. There is also a genuine sympathy for others, which is missing in Pulsatilla. Sleep may be disturbed due to an overactive mind, and even when it occurs it does not refresh.

There is a time aggravation from 1–6 p.m. and a fear of the dark. Discharges are thick, acrid and foul-smelling. Symptoms are usually < undressing. Perspiration is profuse and offensive.

Desire or aversion for foods covers salt, milk, eggs, chocolate, fat and fruit, and the type may swing from one extreme to the other over time. The appetite can be capricious. Like Tuberculinum, there is a craving for foods that aggravate generally.

In the mouth there are ulcers with painful gums, teeth and palate. There are feelings of abdominal tightness and flatulence, and burning pains that are > bending forwards. The motions tend to be hard and there is constipation, with no attempt to pass the stool.

The cough is dry and aggravated by either cold air or a warm room, and talking can also trigger it. Catarrhal conditions of a recurrent nature involving the sinuses and recurrent bronchitis will often respond. There is enlargement of the tonsils, and bleeding from the lungs may also be seen.

There is twitching of muscles, with weakness, especially in thighs. Swelling and pain in legs which is > heat, gentle movement and < brisk movement.

Libido is increased generally, but there are disturbances of function in both sexes. Normal hormonal activity causes swelling and pain in the mammary glands, but without production of milk.

There is urinary incontinence at night. Protein and blood occur in the urine.

Irritation of the skin without eruptions is seen. Warts occur, especially on the hands and feet (or paws). Wounds are slow to heal, but do not have the infection that is seen in the Syphilinum skin. Bleeding ulcers are part of the picture.

A major indication for its use is a family history of much cancer or other diseases with a strong syphilitic component such as tuberculosis. Prolonged childhood illness, especially glandular fever or other illness of viral origin, also calls for its use, and 'never well since' whooping cough or pneumonia is a significant aetiology. It also has a function in relation to the balancing of endocrine function and may be of use in infertility due to ovarian underactivity, and in diabetes mellitus. It has an indication in cases of chronic inflammation of the mammary glands. Skin problems due to hormonal imbalance in neutered animals may also respond. Longstanding grief as an aetiology is found in the picture. It is also useful for the ill effects of vaccination and is often underestimated in this regard. If pain is present it is usually intense. There are similarities in the remedy picture with Nitric Acid.

Scirrhinum

Scirrhinum is one of the preparations originally developed by Compton Burnett. Although classed by some authorities as synonymous with Carcinosin, it is in fact a separate nosode with a different source material, namely tissue from a carcinoma of the liver. In contrast, Carcinosin is prepared using tissues from a mammary carcinoma. While there are many similarities between the two there are also some differences. The fears of Scirrhinum are more marked than those of Carcinosin. Patients are usually thin and chilly, with a marked desire for cold drinks. There is a particular affinity for glands, with stony hardness being a feature of those affected (Ramakrishnan and Coulter, 2001). As well as mammary growths, it also has indications in malignancies of the lungs and liver. It may also be indicated where non-glandular tissues are involved, but again one of the guiding features is extreme hardness. Night-time pains are even more pronounced than with Carcinosin, and there is the tendency to aggravation between 5–6 p.m. It has similarities to Phosphorus in its general modalities (Ramakrishnan, 2001).

The Bowel Nosodes

The bowel nosodes are a group of eleven remedies, developed from the faecal cultures of patients with chronic disease who were responding to treatment. They were developed in the first half of the twentieth century, before the advent and widescale use of antibiotics. In addition to the improvement seen in the presenting picture and the patient's general state of wellbeing, the successful treatments were accompanied by the appearance in the motions of certain specific bacteria. Most of these had the common feature of being essentially gram-negative and none had the ability to ferment lactose; further differentiation was determined by more individual reactions to three other sugars, namely glucose, saccharose and dulcitol.

Which particular bacteria were produced depended on the exact homeopathic remedy that had been administered, but it was found that the same bacteria would be produced in every case when that same remedy was selected correctly as being the simillimum. Eleven groups of bacteria were finally identified, and it was also established that certain remedies would consistently stimulate the appearance of the same group. Each of these bacterial groups has subsequently been used as the source material for one of the remedies known collectively as the bowel nosodes. The other homeopathic remedies whose administration is known to cause the appearance of the appropriate bacteria have been listed and are known, in relation to the bowel nosodes, as associated remedies. Some of these remedies have particularly strong associations, and are hence referred to as leading remedies of the appropriate group, whilst other remedies have a less definite link.

The bowel nosodes are Morgan Pure, Morgan Gaertner, Proteus, Dysentery Co., Faecalis, Mutabile, Sycotic Co., Bacillus No. 7, Bacillus No. 10, Gaertner Bach and Coccal Co. Morgan Pure and Morgan Gaertner are often used together as the remedy Morgan Bach.

The bacteria are produced as a result of a curative action within the body, having been brought about by the administration of the correct homeopathic remedy. The remedy will have been selected by reference to the symptoms being exhibited by the patient, i.e. by reference to the disease process. Hence the remedy produced from the bacteria (the bowel nosode) will also be homeopathic for the disease. Each one has its own remedy picture on which it can be prescribed, but, because of their connection with chronic disease, they can be used in a broader way in its treatment.

The relationship with chronic disease inevitably raises the question of their connection with the miasms. Although the bowel nosodes are not miasmatic remedies in the same way as the others discussed in this chapter, nevertheless it is possible to discern some definite chemical and miasmatic patterns within the groupings of the associated remedies, and hence to identify the miasmatic influences of the bowel nosodes themselves.

Morgan Pure has many associated remedies containing carbon and the carbonates, and as such the psoric miasm is strongly represented there, as it is in the more commonly used Morgan Bach. There is also, however, a definite sycotic element in both, as exemplified by the warts found in the Calc. Carb. picture, the lipomas seen with Baryta Carb. and the strong position of Medorrhinum in the associated remedies of Morgan Pure. Bacillus No. 7 also features in the psoric picture with its keynote of exhaustion and the presence of many Kali remedies in its group. Proteus and Sycotic Co. are predominantly sycotic, with many remedies, such as Thuja and Sepia, showing a connection with water and damp in their pictures.

Gaertner Bach is essentially syphilitic, with its leading associated remedies of Silica, Mercury, and Phosphorus. Dysentery Co. shows both sycotic and syphilitic tendencies in equal degree, with painful abdominal conditions generally and the usefulness of its leading associated remedy Arsenicum Album in the treatment of cancer. The fluorine found in many remedies of the Bacillus No. 10 group gives it a syphilitic bias. Coccal Co. is closely linked to Tuberculinum, although in the context of the basic miasms it is essentially syphilitic, with its emphasis on infection and sepsis.

Consideration of the miasmatic characteristics of the bowel nosodes can be another useful aid to both remedy selection and case management, and the following broad classification should be borne in mind.

PSORA	*Bacillus No. 7*; *Morgan Gaertner*; **Morgan Pure**
SYCOSIS	Bacillus No. 7; Bacillus No. 10; Coccal Co.; *Dysentery Co.*; *Faecalis*; *Morgan Pure*; *Mutabile*; **Proteus**; **Sycotic Co.**
SYPHILIS	Bacillus No. 7; *Bacillus No. 10*; *Dysentery Co.*; *Coccal Co.;* **Gaertner Bach**

CASE 14: *A clear picture of miasmatic influence*

An eight-year-old entire golden retriever was referred because of a persistent and generalised pruritis. There had been no significant illness or drug reactions until the age of five, when the current problems had started. It was known that his sire had died of what was described by the owners as a 'generalised cancer', but there was no other family history. Shortly before the onset of the condition the owner's father had died, which had produced an upset in the family, and the dog had been put in kennels for the only time in his life. Shortly after coming out he developed an abscess on his muzzle, which was lanced under general anaesthetic, and antibiotics were administered as a routine. The abscess resolved but then he began to chew around the base of his tail. He was prescribed topical corticosteroid, followed by systemic steroids as the condition spread.

This pattern continued for two years as the irritation spread over the whole body, and interdigital cysts appeared on the front feet. Over this time there was periodic emptying of the anal glands and several courses of steroids and antibiotics. After two years a lump developed on the outer toe of the left front leg. The toe was removed and histopathology diagnosed a benign tumour. Since then there had been on regular injections of long-acting steroids, which only controlled the pruritis for around two weeks rather than the four weeks which is the more usual clinical experience with this formulation of drug. After two weeks the irritation would begin to return and build up to its maximum over four to five days. The steroid would be administered again at that time. The last injection had been given some four and a half weeks prior to the homeopathic consultation, the owners having decided to pursue a different approach.

On examination there was little visible on the skin except a general dryness and a slight redness. The owner reported that the earflaps occasionally became hot but that there was no discernible pattern and no otitis externa.

The dog was described as highly-strung and sensitive to the moods of those around him. He was easily disciplined and travelled well. He liked much fuss and attention and was friendly to people, although initially a bit wary of strange men. He was wary of noises such as lorries with air brakes but had no fear of thunder or fireworks. He could be aggressive with other dogs. He was a fussy eater with no real interest in food, but preferred what he did eat to be moist rather than dry. He would not eat vegetables and liked cheese, milk and eggs. He would have a good drink at one time. He liked some heat but would pant easily on a hot day and preferred to be outside if possible, in all conditions. He had never learned to cock his leg properly and squatted to pass water.

The appearance of the skin, with no lesions, and the history of neoplasia in both the patient and his sire directed the choice of remedy, and treatment was started with Carcinosin LM1 night and morning for five days. Three weeks later the owner reported a sixty percent improvement in the condition, which improvement had now ceased but not regressed. The dryness in the coat was less, as was the irritation, but the redness could still be seen. The dose of Carcinosin was repeated for two days with no further improvement in the condition. In view of the persisting redness, Sulphur 30c was administered night and morning for three days. This produced a further slight improvement, with the redness disappearing, and the coat quality generally being better, but the pruritis was remained. The Carcinosin LM1 was repeated night and morning for four days, resulting in resolution of the pruritis. This was maintained for three months without further treatment, when a moderate recurrence responded to Carcinosin LM2 given night and morning for four days. There has been no further relapse.

Discussion

The presenting picture, together with the general and family history, pointed to Carcinosin as a possible remedy in its own right. The timing of the onset following the upset in the family was important, but it seemed unlikely that this was a specific case of grief, calling for remedies like Ignatia or Natrum Muriaticum, as there was no overt evidence of a particular bond between the dog and his owner's father. It seemed to be rather an expression of his general sensitivity to the upset in the household at the time, with his being put into kennels also being part of that. The fact that suppression of skin symptoms had led to the appearance of a neoplasm, albeit benign and therefore predominantly sycotic, was considered significant when added to the known family history and led to the use of Carcinosin as a first prescription. The further fact that the initial action of the Carcinosin ceased after a good early response called for either a change of potency, or the possibility of an obstacle to cure and the use of another remedy. The long-term use of the steroids had to be considered as a possible source of the block. A tautological approach using cortisone in potency could have been followed, but Sulphur was decided on as it has uses as a clearing remedy, as well as the local indications pointing to it. It is unusual that a remedy unblocked the action of a nosode rather than the other way round, and hence the action was probably of a clearing nature.

Another consideration is that Sulphur is regarded by Ortega as being more miasmatically balanced than is often supposed. However, the fact that the initially chosen remedy, a miasmatic nosode, was the one that ultimately cleared the condition is an indication of the strong miasmatic nature running through the case. Although it is pure speculation, in the author's opinion further suppressive treatment would almost inevitably have resulted in the appearance of a malignancy in this dog.

CASE 15: *Synergistic effect*

A nine-year-old entire German shepherd dog was suffering from chronic degenerative radiculomyelopathy (CDRM). This first manifested at six years of age as a painless hind leg weakness with incoordination. This increased steadily, and both pedal and patella reflexes became progressively reduced bilaterally. Radiography of the hips and lumbar region revealed no bony abnormalities of clinical significance. Treatment with a range of non-steroidal anti-inflammatory drugs had given no improvement and the owner sought homeopathic treatment.

At the initial homeopathic consultation the dog was only able to rise with difficulty, and was unable to stand for more than a few minutes. Even slight pressure on the lower spine would cause him to collapse on the rear end and sit down. On movement there was a loss of spatial awareness with the hind legs crossing as he walked, and attempting to turn caused him to fall over at the hindquarters. He was fully continent with both faeces and urine.

Apart from the rear end his only other clinical problem was recurring otitis externa, which could involve either ear, but never both together.

The acute attacks of this seemed to be triggered by damp weather, and the discomfort of it was < night. During the attacks there was little discharge but great pain and a putrid smell. He was the dominant dog of three in the household, although essentially tolerant, and was regarded as a 'benevolent dictator'. Appetite and thirst were described as 'normal', and he had always eaten everything that he had been offered. He was friendly to people he knew, but reserved with strangers. He would enjoy attention and petting, and would sometimes ask for it. There was no fear of noise. Mentally he did not appear to be affected by his condition. There was no clear heat desire or aversion.

Initial treatment was with Conium 6c night and morning for ten days, on the indication of ascending paralysis. This produced a strengthening of the hind legs, but with no effect on the ataxia or reflexes. Conium 30c produced no further improvement, but the strength remained. Sulfonal has in its picture staggering gait, reduction of reflexes and weakness in the limbs. It was administered in the 6c night and morning for five days and resulted in an improvement of the condition by about twenty percent. Because the pathology in CDRM is essentially syphilitic, involving demyelination, Syphilinum 200c night and morning for three days was then given, followed by a repeat of the Sulfonal at 30c. This resulted in a significant all-round improvement, which was maintained for two months before deteriorating again. Further doses of Sulfonal at 30c restored the situation.

The case was then maintained on Sulfanol 30c as appropriate. If this failed to act, three doses of Syphilinum 200c were given over a twenty-four hour period, which restored the progress. The attacks of otitis became less frequent and responded to Hepar Sulphuris and Silica. Death occurred from natural causes some four and a half years later.

Discussion

From the miasmatic perspective, demyelination of the nerves is a destructive process, but the symptoms in this case also involved psora. There is also the syphilitic characteristic in the ears of < night. This is a classic example of the nosode, while not completely correcting the basic miasmatic imbalance of a dominant syphilitic influence, reducing and holding it at bay, thereby allowing another remedy to exert its full effect and address the other influences in the case. The Sulfanol was prescribed on the presenting picture of hind limb ataxia, imbalance, reduced reflex action and the painless nature of the hind limb condition. It should be noted that the otitis also improved under the influence of the nosode. The remedies which were prescribed successfully for this, based on more local symptoms, both have significant syphilitic components. Sulfonal, with its symptoms of dysfunction and profound weakness, is essentially a psoric remedy, although chorea and extreme mental irritability (not seen in this case) point to some sycotic influence.

Bibliography

Adler, U.C. (2005) The influence of childhood infections and vaccination on the development of atopy: a systematic review of the direct epidemiological evidence. *Homeopathy* **94,** 182–195

Ageeva, T.K. and Ageev, S.L. (1997) *Modern Homeopathic Therapeutics.* Rossiysky Salon, Moscow

Agrawal, Y.R. (1995) *A Treatise on the Bowel Nosodes.* Vijay Publications, Delhi

Allen, H.C. (1910) *Materia Medica of the Nosodes with X-Ray Provings.* (Reprinted 1982, B. Jain Publishers, New Delhi)

Allen, J.H. (1908) *The Chronic Miasms: Psora and Pseudo-psora.* Privately published in Chicago. (Reprinted 1994, B. Jain Publishers, New Delhi)

Anshutz, E.P. (1900) *New, Old and Forgotten Remedies* (2nd edn 1917). (Reprinted 1993, B. Jain Publishers, New Delhi)

Armstrong, S.E. (2003) Personal communication

Assilem, M.A. (1996) *The Mad Hatter's Tea Party* (2nd edn). Homeopathic Supply Co., Holt, Norfolk. Also Idolatry Inc., California

Azambuja, R.S. (2004) Ontogenesis of the disease. *Cultura Homeopatica* **9**, October issue

Bach, E. (1933) The rediscovery of psora. *British Homeopathic Journal*, April issue

Bach, E. and Wheeler, C.E. (1925) *Chronic Disease. A Working Hypothesis.* (Reprinted 1987, B. Jain Publishers, New Delhi)

Banerjea, S.K. (1993) *Miasmatic Diagnosis.* B. Jain Publishers, New Delhi

Banerjee, P.N. (1931) *Chronic Disease. Its Cause and Cure* [Translation of Ghatak, N., Bengali edition]. B. Jain Publishers, New Delhi

Beattie, N. (1999) Personal communication

Bellavite, P. and Signorini, A. (2002) *The Emerging Science of Homeopathy.* North Atlantic Books, Berkeley, California

Bernard, H. (1950) La reticulo-endothéliose chronique ou sycose. Coquemard, Angoulême, France

Blasig, T. and Vint, P. (2001) *Remedy Relationships.* (English edn trans.

P. Edmonds and H. Waldbaum). Hahnemann Institut, Greifenberg, Germany

Blass, G. (1992) Demystifying the miasms. *British Homeopathic Journal* **82**, 3 (letter)

Burnett, C.J. (1897) *Vaccinosis and its Cure by Thuja: with Remarks on Homoeoprophylaxis*. Homeopathic Publishing Co., London. (Indian edn 1992, B. Jain Publishers, New Delhi)

Chambers (1959) *Twentieth Century Dictionary*. (Revised edn by Geddie, W.)

Chlebowski, R.T. et al (2003) Influence of oestrogen plus progestin on breast cancer and mammography in healthy postmenopausal women. *Journal of the American Medical Association* **289**(3), 3243–3253

Choudhury, H. (1992) *Indications of Miasms*. B. Jain Publishers, New Delhi

Clarke, J.H. (1893) *Therapeutics of the Serpent Poisons*. (Indian edn 1995, B. Jain Publishers, New Delhi)

Clarke, J.H. (1925) *Dictionary of Practical Materia Medica* (3rd edn). (3 vols) Homeopathic Publishing Company, London

Cole, J. and Dyson, R. (1997) *Classical Homeopathy Revisited*. Winter Press, West Wickham, Kent

Coulter, C.R. (1986–98) *Portraits of Homeopathic Medicines*, Vols 1–3. North Atlantic Books, Berkeley, California

Coulter, H.L. (1987) *Aids and Syphilis, the Hidden Link*. North Atlantic Books, Berkeley, California

Cummings, S. (1978) History and development of the bowel nosodes. *Journal of Homeopathic Practice* **1**(2), 78–90

Day, C.E.I. (1990) *Homeopathic Treatment of Small Animals*. C.W. Daniel Company, Saffron Walden, Essex

Dodds, W.J. (1994) Nutritional influences on immune and thyroid function. *American Holistic Veterinary Medical Association Conference* 1994. Orlando, Florida

Dudgeon, R.E. (1853) *Lectures on the Theory and Practice of Homoeopathy*. (Reprinted 1987, B. Jain Publishers, New Delhi)

Duval, D. and Giger, U. (1996) Vaccine associated immune-mediated haemolytic anaemia in dogs. *International Journal of Veterinary Medicine* **10**, 290–295

Elliott, M. (1996) Possible inheritance of miasms. *British Association of Homeopathic Veterinary Surgeons Newsletter*, Spring edition

Elmiger, J. (1998) *Rediscovering Real Medicine*. Element Books, Shaftesbury, Dorset

Evans, M. (1996) Medorrhinum Americana. A proving. *Prometheus Unbound*, Spring issue

Feldman, M. (1996) *Repertory of the Bowel Nosodes*. B. Jain Publishers, New Delhi

Finnegan, M.J.B. (1988) Cyclosporin: simillimum for AIDS? *British Homeopathic Journal* **77**, 215–218

Fortier-Bernovillie, M. (1934) *Syphilis and Sycosis*. (Reprinted 1993, trans. R.K. Mukerji. B. Jain Publishers, New Delhi)

Foubister, D.M. (1954) Clinical impressions of Carcinosin. *British Homeopathic Journal* **44**, April

Francois-Flores, F.D. (2005) *Proceedings of the 60th LIGA Congress*. Berlin

Fraser, P. (2002) *The Aids Miasm*. Winter Press, West Wickham, Kent

Gregory, P.A. (2003) Personal communication

Gutman, W. (1962) Influenza and influenzosis. *British Homeopathic Journal* **51**, 20

Haehl, R. (1922) *Samuel Hahnemann. His Life and Work*. (1992 edn trans. by M.L. Wheeler and W.H.R. Grundy. B. Jain Publishers, New Delhi)

Hahnemann, C.F.S. (1828) *The Chronic Diseases. Their Peculiar Nature and their Homoeopathic Cure*. (Trans. L.H. Tafel 1896 from the 2nd edn, 1835. Reprinted 1978, B. Jain Publishers, New Delhi)

Hahnemann, C.F.S. (1842) *Organon of the Medical Art*, 6th edn. (Trans. Stephen Decker, ed. Wenda Brewster O'Reilly. Birdcage Books, Redmond, California). [Lesser writings. Trans. and ed. 1852 Dudgeon. R.E. Headland, London, and 1993 B. Jain Publishers, New Delhi]

Hallamaa, R.E. et al (2001) Treatment of equine summer eczema with an autogenous serum preparation. *Zeitschrift für Onkologie* **33**, 57–62

Hamilton, D. (1990) *Homeopathic Care for Cats and Dogs*. North Atlantic Books, Berkeley, California

Handley, R. (1997) *In Search of the Later Hahnemann*. Beaconsfield Publishers, Beaconsfield, Buckinghamshire

Hays, J. et al (2003) Effects of estrogen plus progestin on health– related quality of life. *New England Journal of Medicine* **348**(19)

Henneman, K. (1996) Chronic disease and miasms in the horse. *Proceedings of the American Holistic Veterinary Medical Association Conference*, 1996, 148–161

Irwin, M.K.S. (1988) Acquired immunodeficiency syndrome. *British Homeopathic Journal* **77**, 219–223

Johnson, W.M. (1990) *Introduction to Sycosis: its Importance as a Miasm*. B. Jain Publishers, New Delhi

Kent, J.T. (1932) *Lectures on Homoeopathic Philosophy* (4th edn). Boericke and Tafel, Philadelphia

Koehler, G. (1986) *Handbook of Homeopathy*. Thorsons Publishing Group (First published 1983 in Germany as *Lehrbuch der Homöopathie*)

Leary, B. (1990) Psora and history. *British Homeopathic Journal* **79**, 3

Lilley, D. (2005) British Association of Homeopathic Veterinary Surgeons Conference, Bristol

Marim, M. (2003) *Carcinosin – A Clinical Study*. mmarin@ dglnet.com.br

Master, F.J. (1992) *Tubercular Miasm*. B. Jain Publishers, New Delhi

Miles, M. (1992) *Homeopathy and Human Evolution*. Winter Press, West Wickham, Kent

Million Women Study (2003) Breast cancer and hormone replacement. Collaborators' therapy in the million women study. *Lancet* **362**, 419–427

Mondal, T.C. (1998) *Spirit of the Organon, Part 1*. B. Jain Publishers, New Delhi

Murphy, R. (2000) *Homeopathic Remedy Guide*. Hahnemann Academy of North America Press 1996. (Originally published as *The Lotus Materia Medica of Homeopathic and Spagyric Medicines* 1995)

Norland, M. (2003) *Signatures, Miasms, Aids – Spiritual Aspects of Homeopathy*. Yondercott Press, Cullompton, Devon

Ortega, P.S. (1977) *Notes on the Miasms*. (Trans. H. Coulter 1980). National Homeopathic Pharmacy, New Delhi

Paterson, J. (1933) Sycosis and Sycotic Co. *British Homeopathic Journal* **23**, April, 160

Paterson, J. (1936) The role of the bowel flora in chronic disease. *Proceedings of the British Homeopathic Society*, March. (Published in the *British Homeopathic Journal*, April)

Paterson, J. (1949) The bowel nosodes. *British Homeopathic Journal* **40**, 3 July 1950. (Also available as a booklet by A. Nelson & Co., London)

Ramakrishnan, A.U. (2001) *Homeopathic Professionals Teaching Group Masterclass*, Oxford

Ramakrishnan, A.U. and Coulter, C.R. (2001) *A Homeopathic Approach to Cancer*. Ninth House Publishing, Berkeley Springs, California

Reyner, J.H. et al (2001) *Psionic Medicine*. C.W. Daniel Co., Saffron Walden, Essex

Robbins, P. (2004) *Evolving Homeopathy: towards a developmental model for homeopathy*. Privately published, p_robbins@optusnet.com.au

Roberts, H.A. (1936) *The Principles and Art of Cure by Homeopathy*. B. Jain Publishers, New Delhi

Rogers, G. (1963) *'Brother Surgeons'. The Lives of the Hunter Brothers*. Transworld Publishers, London

Rosenthal, C. (2000) Kingdoms understanding in homeopathy – a new approach. *Homeopathic Links*, Issue 1

Rost, A. and Rost, J. (1986) The miasms in contact thermography. *British Homeopathic Journal* **75**(2), 102–112

Sankaran, P. (1978) *Some Notes on the Nosodes*. Homeopathic Medical Publishers, Mumbai

Sankaran, R. (1994) *The Substance of Homoeopathy*. Homeopathic Medical Publishers, Mumbai

Sankaran, R. (1997) *The Soul of Remedies*. Homeopathic Medical Publishers, Mumbai

Saxton, J.G.G. (1994) Bowel nosodes in animals. *Proceedings of the AVHMA Congress*, Orlando, Florida

Saxton, J.G.G. (2000) Suppression – medical crime for the 21st century. *LIGA Conference*, Budapest

Saxton, J.G.G. (2004) *Proceedings of the Faculty of Homeopathy Congress*, Newcastle-upon Tyne

Saxton, J.G.G. (2005) Do we truly understand vaccine reactions and vaccinosis? *Homeopathy* **94**, 200–201

Saxton, J.G.G. and Gregory, P.A. (2005) *Textbook of Veterinary Homeopathy*. Beaconsfield Publishers, Beaconsfield, Buckinghamshire

Schairer, C. et al (2000) Menopausal oestrogen and oestrogen–progestin replacement therapy and breast cancer. *Journal of the American Medical Association* **283**(4), 485–491

Scheffer, M. (1986) *Bach Flower Therapy. Theory and Practice*. Thorsons Publishing Group, Wellingborough, Northamptonshire

Scheibner, V. (2000) *Behavioural Problems in Childhood. The Link to Vaccination*. Australian Print Group, Victoria, Australia

Scholten, J. (1996) *Homeopathy and the Elements*. Stichting Alonnissos, Utrecht, The Netherlands

Schroyens, F. (2004) *Synthesis*, Edition 9.1. Homeopathic Book Publishers, London

Sherr, J.Y. (1992) *The Homeopathic Proving of Hydrogen*. Dynamis, Malvern, Worcestershire

Sherr, J.Y. (2002) *Dynamic Materia Medica – Syphilis*. Dynamis, Malvern, Worcestershire

Sonnenschmidt, R. (2002) Lecture on avian homeopathy. *Handout*, British

Association of Homeopathic Veterinary Surgeons Conference, Harper Adams College, Shropshire

Speight, P. (1977) *Comparison of the Chronic Miasms*. Health Science Press, Saffron Walden, Essex

Squire, B. (1996) *Repertory of Homeopathic Nosodes and Sarcodes*. B. Jain Publishers, New Delhi (Revised edn 1999)

Srinivasulu, G. (2005) Combating epidemics through miasmatic prescription. *Proceedings of the 60th LIGA Congress*, Berlin

Strange, M. (1988) Aids; some early experience. *British Homeopathic Journal* **77**, 224–227

Subramanian, R. (2001) *Miasms. Their Effects on the Human Organism*. B. Jain Publishers, New Delhi

Swayne, J. (ed.) (2000) *International Dictionary of Homeopathy*. Churchill Livingstone, Edinburgh

Teixeira, M.Z. (2002) Is there scientific evidence that suppression of acute diseases in childhood induces chronic disease in the future? *Homeopathy* **91**, 207–216

Tyler, M.L. (1933) *Hahnemann's Conception of Chronic Disease as Caused by Parasitic Micro-organisms*. John Bale & Danielsson, London. Reprinted B. Jain Publishers, New Delhi

van der Zee, H. (2001) *Miasms in Labour*. Stichting Alonnissos, Utrecht, The Netherlands

Vermeulen, F. (1997) *Concordant Materia Medica*. Emryss BV, Haarlem, The Netherlands

Viljoen, A. (1991) Personal communication

Vithoulkas, G. (1980) *The Science of Homeopathy*. Grove Press, New York

Watson, I. (1991) *A Guide to the Methodologies of Homeopathy*. Cutting Edge Publications, Kendal, Cumbria

Whitmont, E.C. (1980) *Psyche and Substance, Essays on Homeopathy in the Light of Jungian Philosophy*. North Atlantic Books, Berkeley, California

Wolff, H.G. (1984) *Homeopathic Medicine for Dogs*. Thorsons Publishers Ltd., Wellingborough, Northamptonshire

Yasgur, J. (1998) *Homeopathic Dictionary and Holistic Health Reference* (4th edn). Van Hoy Publishers, Greenville, Pennsylvania

INDEX